MW01282616

Certified Outpatient Coder (COC™) Exam Study Guide 2019 Edition

Medical Coding Pro

ISBN: 9781794608573

DEDICATION

To the hard working students preparing for the certification exam. Your work ethic and dedication to the medical industry will ensure its health and competency for years to come!

SAVE $50! Use Coupon Code "SAVE50"

The Medical Coding Certification Prep Course

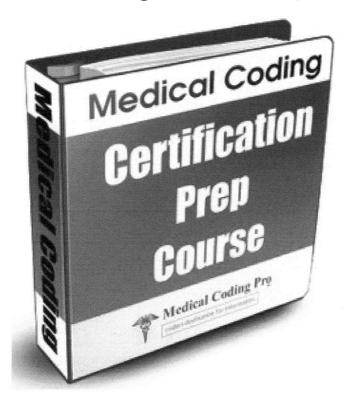

The Medical Coding Certification Prep Course is a web based, self paced, course with over 100 hours of study material. It includes over 700 practice exam questions and answers, 120 Operative Reports, 1,200 terms defined plus current and previous year CPT codes. The course also includes a complete ICD-10 video instruction module, course workbook and one year online access. Professional AAPC approved CPC, CPC-H instructor available to answer questions and give guidance.

For more information go to:

www.MedicalCodingPro.com/medical-coding-certification-prep-course

Quick Start Guide 5

Medical Coding Exam Strategy 6

Overview..16

COC Mock Exam - 150 Questions..20

COC Mock Exam - Answers 100

Scoring Sheets 125

Secrets To Reducing Exam Stress 149

Common Anatomical Terminology 176

Medical Terminology Prefix, Root, and Suffixes....................181

Notes 194

Resources..195

Quick Start Guide

Start by reviewing everything included inside the exam study guide. Contents include the following:

1) Medical Coding Exam Strategy
2) Mock Practice Exam Questions & Answers
3) Scoring Sheets
4) Secrets To Reducing Exam Stress
5) Common Anatomical Terminology
6) Medical Terminology Prefixes, Roots, and Suffixes
7) Notes
8) Resources

These resources will give you a good base to prepare for the board exam.

If you have any questions please email contact us at support@medicalcodingpro.com.

Medical Coding Exam Strategy

One of the first things we should discuss is what "The Strategy" is and what it isn't.

What it is:

A simple, yet powerful, method for increasing your chances of passing the certification exam. Many people have told us that time management was their biggest obstacle in passing the exam. This is what "The Strategy" addresses. It is a road map to pass the exam. It has very little to do with coding knowledge and everything to do with your approach.

What it isn't:

A long, drawn out, hard to follow maze with do's and don'ts reviewing the material that was covered in class. We assume that you know the material, otherwise, it doesn't matter what we teach you the odds are against you.

Why it is important: The reality is many people do not pass the exam the first time. This becomes a costly proposition and one that wasn't bargained for because the next step is an exam retake. The cost: $380. Some even go further and sign up for a three day "boot camp". The cost: about $1200.

Between a rock and a hard place

In this very typical example you passed the Medical Coding class with flying colors but the major hospitals and doctor offices all want a certified medical coder. Why, because it increases their output, makes them more money, and limits their liability for mistakes. So now you're stuck. You have to get certified, but at what cost? It all depends how many times you have to take the certification exam. Follow the steps outlined in "The Strategy" and your next exam could reward you with a certification.

Start by reviewing common mistakes

Some of the most common mistakes made while taking the exam are what we like to call "time wasters". The most important factor to succeeding is time management. You only have 5 hours and 40 minutes to complete the exam (including breaks) and it consists of 150 questions so every minute counts.

The time breakdown goes like this: Exam Time (without breaks) 5 hours 40 minutes or 340 minutes. Exam length: 150 Questions. The easy math is two minute per question. What can we eliminate to save time?

Things Not To Do

1) Answer each question in numerical order.
2) Take too much time on difficult questions first.
3) Read the doctors chart before reading the detail of the question.
4) Not highlighting questions "passed" in the first round

Time Waster #1:

Answering each question in numerical order

If you answer each question in numerical order you will never finish the exam! This is one of the most common mistakes made. If you start out answering the first several questions just fine and then ten questions into the exam you come to a one that you have trouble with, what then? This is a "time burner" and one you can not get hung up on. We will review why this is more important later in "The Strategy".

The Exam is five hours and forty minutes and 150 questions... an average of two minutes per question. The key is to redistribute your time.

Time Waster #2:

Taking too much time on difficult questions the first time through the exam

"The Strategy" is based on a "two pass" system. The first pass is designed to answer the easy questions and highlight the more difficult ones. These will be addressed on the second pass. A good rule of thumb is if you can't answer it in a minute and a half, move on! If you continue to work on these questions you run the risk of not completing the exam or having to rush through the more difficult questions at the end.

Time Waster #3:

Reading the doctors chart before reading the detail of the question

If you get caught in this "time waster" it will rob you of valuable minutes. Always read the question completely before reading the doctors chart. You may be able to eliminate much of the chart because the question is requesting limited information or specific detail.

Time waster #4:

Not highlighting the more difficult questions for the second "pass"

Be prepared. Have a game plan and stick to it. Make sure that you highlight the more difficult questions that you are going to "pass" on in the first round of the exam. If you make the mistake of not highlighting these questions, you will lose valuable minutes trying to search for them in the second round.

Your goal is to answer the easier questions in a minute and a half maximum! Out of 150 questions, let's assume you can answer 60%, or 90 questions, on the first pass averaging 1 minutes per question. That is a total of 135 minutes to answer the first 90 questions. Again, this is an average. That leaves you with 165 minutes to answer the remaining 60 questions. That comes out to 2 minutes per question on the second pass! Now you can be more deliberate with the remaining, more difficult, questions to make sure you answer them correctly.

The "time wasters" have to be minimized or eliminated for you to be successful. Every minute you can save on looking up codes or moving more difficult questions to the second pass the closer you are to your certification.

"Time Wasters" have to be avoided at all costs. Implement a "two pass" system and watch your results increase substantially!

Now let's take an in depth look at the keys that will make all the difference in your exam experience. These are "The Strategy" and "The "Keys" to passing a certification exam! These are not difficult, complex strategies. These are straight forward, simple strategies that are easy to implement and highly effective. Follow each step and you will be well on your way to certification.

The Exam Strategy:

1) The basic element of the strategy is making two passes through the exam. The first pass is to answer the questions you can complete in 1 . minute or less. This should be about 60% of the questions. If you can not answer a question in that time, highlight it (mark it for the second pass) and move on! That creates 2 minutes for the remaining 40% which you have identified as more difficult. This should leave you plenty of time on the more difficult questions and improve your overall score.

2) Answer the easier questions in each section on the first pass. You have to answer 70% of the questions or better correctly to pass so answering the easier questions in each section will form a good base of correctly answered questions in all sections thus improving your chances of passing.

3) Identify the first three numbers of the code first. This will help you eliminate answers instantly and narrow your choices for the correct answer. This is a big "time saver". Practice this on your mock practice exam.

4) Read each question before reading the entire doctors chart. Another big "time saver"! Don't waste valuable time reading the entire doctors chart before reading the question. Read the entire question first to find out the specific information the question is requesting.

5) Highlight Procedures one color, Diagnosis another color and Modifiers a third color for quick reference (again, a big time saver!)

The Keys to Success:

Key #1: Study and Preparation.

Don't let anyone fool you into thinking that you don't have to study. That is not the case. You NEED to study, and study hard! The Exam Strategy assumes that you know all the material. There are no shortcuts and The Exam Strategy will only help you pass if you know the material. So put in the time!

One of the best tools available to practice time management for the exam is the Medical Coding Exam System

(www.MedicalCodingExamSystem.com).

It is course dedicated strictly to time management. This will pay big dividends during the exam. We also highly the Faster Coder (www.fastercoder.com) to improve your speed and accuracy. You will quickly find it is worth its weight in gold.

Key #2: Two Complete Passes through the Exam.

During the exam you will be making TWO passes through the entire exam. Let me repeat this because it is at the heart of what we are trying to accomplish. During the exam you will be going through the entire exam twice! The first pass is to answer the easier questions and the second pass is to answer the more difficult ones. Many people do not pass the exam because they get caught up on a few difficult questions and end up not completing the entire exam. You must follow this key element as it is your key to success.

Key #3: Answer The First Pass Questions in 1 1/2 Minutes or Less.

Start the exam by making a first pass. During the first pass answer all the questions that you can complete in a reasonable amount of time (1 1/2 minutes). If you can't answer the question in 1 1/2 minutes highlight it and move on!

Key #4: Highlight All Unanswered Questions in First Pass

If you cannot answer a question within 1 1/2 minutes of the first pass, highlight the unanswered questions in yellow for easy reference during the second pass! Do not forget to highlight them as every second counts and this could be a big time saver!

Key #5: Answer the More Difficult Questions during Second Pass

You should complete the first pass in 135 minutes or less. This will establish a good base of answered questions and leave you with 165 minutes or more to go back and answer the highlighted questions.

Key #6: Do Not Answer the Questions in Order, You Will Fail!

If you take your time and answer the first 80% of questions perfect but run out of time and have to guess on the remaining 20% questions, YOU WILL NOT PASS. You must answer 70% of the questions correctly to pass the exam!

Key #7: Identify the First Three Numbers of the Code

Another good "time saver" is to identify the first three numbers of the code, turn to that page, then go to the sub code numbers.

Key #8: You Can Miss a Certain Percentage in each Section

You can miss a certain percentage in each section and still pass the exam. Your goal is to get enough right to pass. Making two complete passes through the exam will ensures that you are, at minimum, answering the easy questions in each section first. This alone will increase your chances of passing because you will have a base of questions answered in each section. Typically, the last section is rushed through. This will eliminate this hurdle.

Key #9: Read Each Question before Reading the Doctors Chart

Go over each question before you read the doctors chart. This will tell you exactly what you are looking for. You may not need to read the entire chart because the question only references a specific section. This will save you precious time.

Key #10: Highlight Procedures, Diagnosis, and Modifiers

Highlight the patient's treatment/s in different colors for easy reference. I recommend using these colors: Yellow for Procedures, Blue for Diagnosis, and Pink for Modifiers.

Key #11: You Must Answer 70% correctly to pass the exam

You must keep moving! Leave the tough questions and move on. Ask around to anyone who did not pass the exam the first time (or more) and see what they say. It's all about time management and using the right tips and techniques. So to that end, if you do not follow any other advice, follow this! Do the easiest questions first.

Bonus Tips:

1) Eliminate any answers that begin with an V-Code instantly! Cross it out... this will reduce your selection of answers.

2) Code injections with an administration charge.

3) Supervision and Interpretation components require physician supervision. In radiology procedures this means the radiologist has participated.

4) Know the difference between modifier 26 and modifier TC from your HCPCS II book.

5) Diabetes mellitus – etiology code first then the manifestation code.

6) Trauma accident- always code the most severe injury first

7) Tab all your books including CPT, HCPCS Level II, ICD-10-CM, for quick reference.

8) Code burns on the depth of the burn (1st, 2nd, or 3rd degree). Burns are classified to the extent of the body surface involved. When coding burns of multiple sites, assign separate codes for each burn site. Also burns of the same local site (three-character category level, T20-T28), but of different degrees should be coded to the highest degree documented.

9) Multiple fractures, code by site and sequence by severity.

10) If the same bone is fractured or dislocated, code the fracture only.

11) If the question doesn't state open or closed fracture, code as a closed fracture.

12) Late effects (now called "sequela); is a residual of previous illness or injury. Code the residual and then the cause. Reference "late" in the index.

13) Sequence symptoms first if no diagnosis.

14) Study Medicare A, B, C, D

15) Understand modifier 62 co-surgeons (look on exam for surgeon A and B)

16) ***KEEP MOVING, KEEP MOVING, AND KEEP MOVING!***

Overview

Certified Outpatient Coder (COC)

Outpatient ambulatory coder jobs are trending faster than ever before. As physicians move away from private practices and join hospital groups, career opportunities in outpatient facilities such as ambulatory surgical centers or hospital outpatient billing and coding departments are opening for coders. The COC™ (formerly CPC-H®) exam validates your specialized payment knowledge needed for these jobs in addition to your CPT®, ICD-10, and HCPCS Level II coding skills. Invest in your future with the COC™ medical coding certification.

Certified COC's abilities in outpatient facility/hospital services include:

• Proficiency in assigning accurate medical codes for diagnoses, procedures and services performed in the outpatient setting (emergency department visits, outpatient clinic visits, same day surgeries, diagnostic testing (radiology and laboratory), and outpatient therapies (physical therapy, occupational therapy, speech therapy, and chemotherapy)

• Proficiency across a wide range of services, including evaluation and management, anesthesia, surgical services, radiology, pathology, and medicine

• Knowledge of coding rules and regulations along with proficiency on issues regarding medical coding, compliance, and reimbursement under outpatient grouping systems. COC's can better handle issues such as medical necessity, claims denials, bundling issues, and charge capture

• Ability to integrate coding and reimbursement rule changes in a timely manner to include updating the Charge Description Master (CDM), fee updates, and the Field Locators (FL) on the UB04

• Correctly completing a CMS 1500 for ASC services and UB04 for outpatient services, including the appropriate application of modifiers

• Knowledge of anatomy, physiology, and medical terminology commensurate with ability to correctly code provider services and diagnoses

• A working knowledge in the assignment of ICD-10-CM codes from Volumes 1 & 2

Note:

ICD-10-PCS and DRG code assignment (inpatient coding) are not tested during the COC exam.

The COC™ Exam

- 150 multiple-choice questions (proctored)

- 5 hours and 40 minutes to finish the exam

- One free retake

- $425 ($325 AAPC Students)

- Open code book (manuals)

The COC™ examination consists of questions regarding the correct application of CPT®, HCPCS Level II procedure and supply codes and ICD-10-CM diagnosis codes used for coding and billing outpatient facility/ hospital and freestanding ASC services to insurance companies.

Exam Requirements

• We recommend having an associate's degree.

• Pay examination fee at the time of application submission.

• Maintain current membership with the AAPC.
◦ New members must submit membership payment with examination application.
◦ Renewing members must have a current membership at the time of submission and when exam results are released.

A COC (formerly CPC-H) must have at least two years medical coding experience (member's with an apprentice designation are not required to have two years medical coding experience.) Membership is required to be renewed annually and 36 Continuing Education Units (CEU's) must be submitted every two years for verification and authentication of expertise.

Mock Practice Exam Questions & Answers

The following is a Medical Coding Pro mock practice exam. You may not use any outside materials for this exam other than the manuals referenced by the American Academy of Professional Coders (AAPC ©).

The code research program we use and recommend is Find A Code. You can locate it at: www.findacode.com?pc=MEDCOPRO.

To pass the certification exam you must manage your time carefully. If after going through this practice you determine that time management is a skill you may need additional assistance with, the Medical Coding Exam System (www.MedicalCodingExamSystem.com) is an excellent resource for additional support.

If you want additional resources to prepare for the certification exam we highly recommend FasterCoder.com (www.FasterCoder.com).

COC Mock Exam - 150 Questions

Medical Terminology - 10 Questions

1. A genioplasty is:

a. Surgical repair and ion of the bony components of the chin
b. Surgical repair and ion of the bony components of the cheekbones
c. Insertion of a plastic prosthesis into the genital area
d. Surgical repair of the genioglossus muscle

2. The reduction of intrathoracic space by removing sections of the chest wall is known as a:

a. Thoracentesis
b. Thoracostomy
c. Thoracotomy
d. Thoracoplasty

3. The obturator nerve is found:

a. In the neck
b. In the thorax
c. In the abdomen
d. In the thigh region

4. Which of the following is NOT a valid somatic nerve?

a. Vagus
b. Axillary
c. Inferior occipital nerve
d. Pudendal

5. Pneumothorax is a:

a. Collapsed lung
b. Disease of the lung
c. Specifically, a type of pneumonia
d. Disease of the throat

6. Enterocystoplasty is a:

a. Repair of the urethra.
b. Repair of the bladder (bladder augmentation)
c. Repair of the ureter.
d. Repair of the kidney or kidneys.

7. Cystorrhaphy

a. Removal of a cyst from the bladder
b. Surgical repair of a defect or wound in the urinary bladder.
c. Repair of the urethra.
d. Creating an opening into the urinary bladder.

8. A strangulated hernia:

a. A reducible hernia.
b. A hernia that impedes the patient's trachea.
c. One that is trapped and cannot return to the abdomen.
d. Although it sounds severe, this is the least dangerous type of hernia.

9. The difference, respectively, between autogenic and autologous is:

a. Antonyms. Originating from within; originating from without
b. Derived from ; Similar to
c. Simple to use; Simple to learn
d. None. They both mean originating from within the body

10. Avulsion means:

a. Destruction by electrical cauterization.
b. Excising via surgical knife.
c. A tearing away or forcible separation.
d. The separation of a donor graft from the host.

Anatomy - 10 Questions

11. Submental

a. Above the chin
b. Larger than average size chin
c. Under the chin
d. Of lower than average intelligence

12. The ethmoid sinus is a:

a. Honeycomb-like structure and is located between the eyes.
b. Star-shaped structure and is located between the ears.
c. V-shaped structure and is located between the eyes.
d. Oval structure and is located just above the frenulum.

13. Which below is NOT one of the functions of the kidneys?

a. Filters blood
b. Regulates blood pressure
c. Eliminates waste
d. None of the answers are correct

14. A frenulum:

a. Is a structure found on the prepuce, clitoris and tongue.
b. Like the frenulum of Morgagni, is named after the Italian pathologist,
    Giovanni B Morgagni.
c. A small frenum or frenula
d. All of the above are correct

15. The Medulla Oblongata is located:

a. At the front of the brain
b. At the back of the brain
c. Just below the pineal gland
d. Just below the pons. It is part of the brain stem

16. Which organ has both exocrine and endocrine parts?

a. Bladder
b. Stomach
c. Kidney
d. Pancreas

17. The parietal bone is:

a. At the base of the skull,
b. The largest bone of the skull, superior to the occipital bone.
c. Anterior to the Frontal bone and Posterior to the occipital bone.
d. The bone on the side of the skull where the ear is.

18. The popliteal area is near where:

a. Neck
b. Armpit
c. Knee
d. Foot

19. The adductor magnus is found:

a. In the Neck
b. In the Outer Thigh
c. In the Inner Thigh
d. In the Buttocks

20. Which of the following is NOT one of the heart valves?

a. Tricuspid
b. Atrial
c. Mitral
d. Pulmonary

Coding Guidelines - 6 Questions

21. DIAGNOSES: 1. Foreign body in right middle ear. 2. Right tympanic membrane perforation.

OPERATION: 1. Myringoplasty with fat patch graft. 2. Removal of right middle ear foreign body.

INDICATIONS: The patient is a 7-year-old who has had three sets of PE tubes placed in the past. Tubes which were placed by myself approximately two years ago have since extruded. He recently developed a middle ear infection with rupture of the tympanic membrane on the right. He has a tympanic membrane perforation on the left which has been stable. After several weeks of drop usage and antibiotics and visualization with the operating microscope (it should be noted the patient is quite difficult to examine because of his lack of cooperation in the office), it appeared he had a foreign body in the middle ear space, which was consistent with an old tube, a type that I do not use, probably from a previous PE tube placement. It was located in the middle ear space with a substantial amount of granulation and inflammation surrounding it.

PROCEDURE: The patient was taken to the operating room and placed in the supine position. After adequate endotracheal anesthesia was obtained, the patient was prepped and draped in a sterile fashion. A postlobular incision was made on the right side to harvest fat from the posterior lobule area of the right ear. This was obtained, and then closure was performed with a 4-0 Monocryl subcutaneous and subcuticular closure. Attention was then directed toward the right ear where the right ear was cleaned of purulent material which was quite evident. There was an anterior perforation, and deep into the middle ear space could be visualized an old tube lying in the middle ear space anteriorly. This was removed using an alligator forceps. The edges of the tympanic membrane perforation were freshened with a Rosen needle. The middle ear space was then thoroughly irrigated with Cortisporin drops. The Gelfoam was placed into the middle ear space medially, and the fat was placed with fat exuding from the middle ear space and filling up the perforation site. Then, Gelfoam was placed lateral to the myringoplasty site.

The patient tolerated the procedure well and returned to the recovery room awake and in stable condition.

a. 69200-RT
b. 69620-RT, 69424-51-RT
c. 69205-RT, 69620-51-RT
d. 69620-RT

22. Level II HCPCS modifiers to identify fingers (and thumbs) are:

a. FA-F9
b. TA-T9
c. P1-P9
d. There are no codes

23. Would MOD-25 be appropriate for billing on the UB-04 form?

a. Yes, use as you would for Pro Fees
b. No, MOD-25 is not an appropriate MOD
c. Yes, but only on type "S" and type "T" procedures
d. It can be used but really doesn't matter, since it does not impact reimbursement

24. Modifier -58 would most likely be used during which of the procedures below?

a. E & M Visits, Emergency Department (99281-99285)
b. Simple skin repairs (codes 12001-12021)
c. Free skin grafts (codes 15271-152780)
d. Transluminal Balloon Angioplasty

25. The X- modifiers:

a. Are new for 2017
b. Replace mod -25
c. Replace mod -59
d. Are not accepted by Medicare.

26. Charging for services that are not medically necessary, do not conform to professionally recognized standards, or are unfairly priced is known as:

a. Fraud
b. Abuse
c. Violation of Stark Laws
d. A HIPAA violation

Compliance - 4 Questions

27. Per HIPAA, a covered entity may, without the individual's authorization, use or disclose protected health information for its own treatment, payment, and health care operations activities.

a. To avoid interfering with an individual's access to quality health care.
b. To avoid interfering with the efficient payment for such health care.
c. With certain limits and protections.
d. All of the answers are correct.

28. What is the role of JCAHO?

a. JCAHO is a government sponsored, mandatory accreditation program for hospitals.

b. JCAHO is part of the Department of Health and Human Services (DHHS)

c. Is a not-for-profit organization which operates, fee-based, accreditation programs to subscriber hospitals and other health-care organizations.

d. Is a private-sector, free, ranking program for hospital accreditation programs.

29. The OIG is made up of ____ components of which ____ is one of those components.

a. 3, Office of Audit Services (OAS)
b. 4, Office of Evaluation and Inspections (OEI)
c. 6, Office of Management and Policy (OMP)
d. 8, Immediate Office of the Inspector General (IO).

30. It is permissible to waive patient co-payments or deductibles:

a. Never.
b. When the patient is an employee of the organization.
c. As long as the clinic or provider makes up the difference.
d. Only for Medicare patients who are unable to pay.

CPT - 22 Questions

31. Code for the removal of a subcutaneous 3 cm tumor from the soft tissue of the right hip.

a. 27043
b. 27043-RT
c. 27047
d. 27047-RT

32. Code for the laparoscopic revision and removal of a prosthetic vaginal graft?

a. 57425
b. 57426
c. 57423
d. 57421

33. Code a goniotomy of both eyes with an ophthalmic endoscope:

a. 65810
b. 65820
c. 65820-50
d. 65820-50, 66990-51

34. What code should be reported to Medicare when performing an E & M Consultation?

a. Use the New Patient Codes
b. Use an unlisted code
c. Consultations cannot be reported. It is a non-billable service.
d. Use the prolonged service E & M Codes

35. A 55-year-old female underwent a total urethrectomy with cystostomy.

a. 53210
b. 53215
c. 51040, 53210-51
d. 51040, 53210-52

36. Code for a colonoscopy of the entire colon, from the rectum to the cecum plus the terminal ileum, with biopsy.

a. 44160
b. 45380-52
c. 45380
d. 45380, 45378-51

37. The difference between morbidity and mortality is:

a. There is no difference. They are synonyms.

b. Morbidity refers to a disease or the incidence of disease within a population while mortality is the death rate as a result of a disease.

c. Morbidity refers to the death rate as a result of a disease while mortality refers to a disease or the incidence of disease within a population.

d. Morbidity refers to the death rate of the population over a certain age while mortality refers to the death rate of the total population.

38. Preventive medicine codes would commonly be used for:

a. Annual check-up
b. Sports physical
c. A "well baby" exam
d. All of the answers are correct

39. Code for the insertion of an implant outside the muscular cone, after evisceration of the ocular contents.

a. 65130
b. 65130, 69990
c. 65135
d. 67550

40. Code for a internal dwelling renal transplantation via snare and the replacement of Internally Dwelling Ureteral Stent via a percutaneous approach.

a. 50380
b. 50382
c. 50384
d. 50387

41. Code for a transanal approach for the excision of a partial thickness rectal tumor:

a. 45160
b. 45171
c. 45172
d. 45190

42. Hospital Discharge Codes 99238 and 99239:

a. Include all E & M services performed on the day of discharge.
b. Do NOT include any E & M services performed on the day of discharge.
c. Include only those E & M services performed by the discharging physician.
d. Are only used when the patient is admitted and discharged on the same day.

43. Mr. Morgenstern, was found to have a right proximal ureteral calculus. Dr. Cooper used a right retrograde pyelogram to reveal the proximal ureteral stone. He performed a cystoscopy with manipulation and ureteral Stent placement. The operation was uneventful and the patient tolerated the procedure well. Code the procedure(s) and the radiological guidance.

a. 52330, 52332
b. 52330, 52332-51
c. 52330, 52332-51, 74400
d. 52330, 52332-51, 74420

44. Locations, valid for critical care are:

a. Coronary care unit
b. Intensive care unit
c. Respiratory care unit
d. All the answers are correct

45. The patient underwent TURP which includes: vasectomy, meatotomy, cystourethroscopy, urethral calibration, and internal urethrotomy. There was a moderate amount of postoperative bleeding which was controlled.

a. 52601
b. 52601, 55250, 53020
c. 52601, 55250, 53020, 52000, 52275
d. 53020, 52000

46. When adding multiple repair sites:

a. Add all of the wounds in the same anatomical site regardless of type.
b. Add all of the same type, regardless of location.
c. Add only same type, same anatomical site grouping (per CPT codes).
d. Add only those of the same approximate size.

47. The physician made three incisions into the necrotic dermis to lessen the constriction of the third degree circumferential burns of both of the patient's arms. Code for this:

a. 16025-RT-LT
b. 16025-50 X 3
c. 16035-50, 16036-50 X 2
d. 16035 X 3

48. Code for ERCP, with destruction of stones by lithotripsy (any method), with endoscopy and sphincterotomy.

a. 43265, 43262
b. 43265, 43262-51-22
c. 43265, 43262-51
d. 43265, 43262-51, 43260-51

49. Code the removal and replacement of a permanent pacemaker, pulse generator only.

a. 33233
b. 33212
c. 33233, 33212-51
d. 33216

50. Report the open endovascular revascularization of the tibial artery, with atherectomy.

a. 37228
b. 37229
c. 37230
d. 37231

51. The physician injected 100ml of Mannitol, a 25% in 50 ml solution. Code for the HCPCS code.

a. J2150
b. J2150 X 2
c. J2175
d. J2180

52. Report the Medicare code for trimming of three dystrophic toenails.

a. G0127
b. G0127 X 3
c. S0390
d. 11719

HCPCS - 8 Questions

53. Code for an enteral nutrition pump with alarm:

a. B5200
b. B9002
c. B9004
d. B9006

54. Code for 120 mg of Myolin:

a. J7517, 90471
b. J7517 X 2, 90471
c. J2360, 90471
d. J2360 X 2, 90471

55. Level II HCPCS modifiers to identify toes are:

a. FA-F9
b. TA-T9
c. P1-P9
d. There are no codes.

56. A non-Medicare patient was given a 1.8 mg injection of Thyrotropin Alfa in the doctor's office. Code for the injection and the administration of the injection.

a. J3240
b. J3240 X 2, 90471
c. J3240 X 2, 90473
d. J3240 X 2, 36415 X 2

57. Code for an IV Toradol injection - 30 mg:

a. J1885 X 2, 96374
b. J1885, 96372
c. J3265, 96374 X 2
d. J3265 X 2

58. Report a bilateral screening mammography, a subsequent Medicare Annual Wellness Exam (AWV) with an established E & M Visit, EPF Hx and Exam and LOW MDM (the CC was GERD and HTN).

a. 99387, G0439, 77067
b. G0439 Only
c. 99213, G0439-33, 77067
d. This is a sick visit so only report 99213 and the 77066 code.

59. A patient received a 12 sq. cm. dermal tissue substitute of human origin, without other bioengineered elements, without metabolically active elements. This treatment was completed due to a burn on the abdomen. How would you report the supply?

a. C1762
b. J7342
c. C1763
d. J7340

60. Modifiers E1, E2, E3 and E4 are:

a. HCPCS modifiers for the toes.
b. HCPCS modifiers for the fingers.
c. HCPCS modifiers for the eyelids
d. CPT modifiers for eyelids.

ICD-10 - 30 Questions

61. Johnny was shot in the back by his friend with a pellet gun while playing in their backyard. The pellet, because of its odd shape, was difficult to extract.

a. S21.209A, Y92.017
b. S31.020A, W34.010A, Y92.79
c. S31.020A, W33.01XA, Y92.838
d. S31.020A, W34.010A, Y92.017

62. The patient has been depressed and unable to sleep for several days. The provider documented in the record: Cluster headache, fibromyalgia, jaw pain, Depression NOS.

a. G44.029, M79.7, R68.84, F32.9
b. G44.009, M79.7, R06.7, F32.9
c. G44.009, R68.84, M79.7, F32.9
d. G44.009, R68.84, F41.8

63. The patient, a 55-year-old male, was a passenger in an automobile accident where the vehicle hit the divider. The patient presents with a crushed skull, cerebral laceration and contusions. The patient was unconscious for 90-minutes and later developed post-traumatic seizures. Which codes best represent this situation?

a. S06.330A, G40.301 V86.09XA
b. S06.333A, V48.6XXA
c. S06.333A, R56.1, V86.19XA
d. S02.0XXA, R56.9, V49.9XXA

64. The patient, a four-year-old child, complained of pain from inside her left ear. The doctor found a retained glass fragment in the child's ear.

a. H74.8X2, Z18.81
b. H92.02, Z18.81
c. H92.02, H74.8X2, Z18.81
d. H92.02, H74.8X2, S00.452A

65. What is the correct sequencing order of the following ICD-10 Codes: Z37.0, O80, O44.03

a. O80, Z37.0, O44.03
b. Z37.0, O80, O44.03
c. Z37.0, O80 assuming the this was a normal delivery without complications.
d. O80, Z37.0, assuming the this was a normal delivery without complications.

66. What is Antineoplastic chemotherapy induced pancytopenia and how do you report it?

a. D61.810, reduction of one's red cell, neutrophil, and platelet count.
b. D61.810, evidenced by anemia, neutropenia, and thrombocytopenia.
c. Both answers (a) and (b) are correct.
d. None of the answers are correct.

67. Code for the following:

1. Left chronic anterior and posterior ethmoiditis.
2. Left chronic maxillary sinusitis with polyps.
3. Left inferior turbinate hypertrophy.
4. Right anterior and posterior chronic ethmoiditis.
5. Right chronic maxillary sinusitis with polyps.
6. Right chronic inferior turbinate hypertrophic.
7. Intranasal deformity causing nasal obstruction due to septal deviation.

a. J32.2, J32.0, J33.9, J34.2
b. J32.2, J32.0, J33.8, J34.3, M95.0
c. J32.2, J32.0, J33.8, J34.3, J34.2
d. J32.9, J32.2, J34.2, J32.0, J33.9, J34.3

68. Code for a myocardial infarction as a result of a complete blockage and define "infarction":

a. It means to plug up. I21.4
b. It means death or "to die". I21.3
c. It means to expand or grow. I21.4
d. It means "inflammation of". I21.3

69. DIAGNOSES: 1. Bilateral chronic serous otitis media. 2. Chronic adenotonsillitis. 3. Adenotonsillar hypertrophy.

a. H66.009, J35.01, J35.02
b. H65.23
c. H65.23, J35.03
d. H65.23, J35.3, J35.01

70. DIAGNOSES: 1. Foreign body in right middle ear. 2. Right tympanic membrane perforation. The foreign body is a ventilating tube placed by another physician.

a. H74.8X9
b. H74.8X1, H72.91
c. H74.8X1, H66.11
d. H74.8X1, S00.05XA

71. An elderly patient falls from her wheelchair in her home and sustains a displaced, compound fracture of the left tibial spine and fibula.

a. S82.112B, W05.0XXA, Y92.019
b. S82.201C, S82.401C
c. S82.101A, W05.1XXA
d. W05.0XXA, Y92.099, S82.109A, S82.839A

72. Code for a return visit for paraplegia from previous laceration of spinal cord injury of the thoracic spine.

a. G82.51
b. G82.20, S14.9XXS
c. G82.20, S24.2XXS
d. G83.89

73. Code for secondary benign hypertension; stenosis of renal artery due to arterial fibromuscular dysplasia , erectile dysfunction following interstitial seed therapy, and a personal history of malignant neoplasm of prostate.

a. I15.0, N52.36, N50.82
b. I77.3, N52.01
c. I15.0, N52.2, R10.30
d. None of the answers are correct.

74. Following a vehicle accident, in which the car was hit by an oncoming SUV on the highway, the patient is brought to the ER to be checked out for injuries. She had hit the steering wheel hard. The patient complains of generalized pain in her chest area. After examination, the physician rules out any heart problems and cannot find any problems and the patient is released.

a. R07.9, Z04.1
b. R07.9, V49.88XA, Y92.410
c. R52, V49.88XA, Y92.410, Z04.3
d. R07.9, V43.51XA, Y92.410, Z04.1

75. 12-year-old female was chasing her friend when she fell through a sliding glass door sustaining three lacerations. Left knee 5.5 cm laceration, involving deep subcutaneous tissue and fascia, was repaired with layered closure using 1% lidocaine anesthetic. Right knee: 7.2 cm laceration was repaired under local anesthetic with a single-layer closure. Right hand: 2.5 cm laceration of the dermis was repaired with simple closure using Dermabond© tissue adhesive.

Assessment: Wounds of both knees and left hand requiring suture repair

Plan: Follow-up in 10 days for suture removal. Call office if any questions or complications. What are the correct ICD-10-CM and CPT procedure codes? Do not code anesthesia administration.

a. S81.012A, S81.011A, S61.411A, W01.110A, Y92.009, 12005
b. S81.012A, S81.011A, S61.411A, 12002-RT, 12032-51-LT, 17999-51-LT
c. S71.009A, 12032, 12002-LT, A4364
d. S81.012A, S81.011A, S61.411A, W01.110A, Y92.099, 12032-LT, 12004-51-RT

76. A patient is seen today for a speech therapy session. He has been experiencing dysarthria following an acute case of viral encephalitis. What code(s) should be reported?

a. Z51.89
b. R47.1, B94.1, Z51.89
c. B94.1
d. B94.1, A17.1

77. The patient, a four-year old child, complained of pain from inside her ear. The doctor found a retained glass fragment in the child's ear.

a. H92.09, H74.8x9, Z18.83
b. H92.09, H74.8x9, Z18.81
c. H92.09, H74.43, Z18.81
d. H92.09, H69.80, Z18.81

78. Code for 1. Hematuria. 2. Chronic Prostatitis. 3. Right ureteral stricture.

a. N20.1, R31.9, N13.5
b. N20.1, N41.1
c. R31.9, N41.1, N13.5
d. N20.1, N13.5, R31.9, N41.1

79. Code for the first encounter and setting of a fracture of the right fibula due to osteogenesis imperfecta.

a. M84.469A, Q78.0
b. M84.463A,
c. S82.839A, Q78.0
d. None of the answers are correct

80. Code for septicemia due to streptococcus:

a. A41.89, B95.3
b. A40.9, B95.0
c. A40.9, B95.3
d. None of the answers are correct.

81. What code(s) are reported for a patient who comes to the emergency room for active treatment of a metal splinter in his left cornea from a drill press where he works in a factory?

a. S05.52XA, Y92.838
b. T15.02XA, W31.1XXA, Y92.63
c. S05.52XA, W31.1XXA, Y92.63
d. T15.00XA, T56.91XA, Z18.10

82. Report constipation due to Oncovin injected for Hodgkin's disease.

a. K59.00, C81.99, Z85.72
b. K59.00, C81.99
c. C85.80
d. K59.00

83. Code for a coma due to combination of prescribed Seconal with alcoholic beverages.

a. F13.20, R40.20
b. F13.20
c. R40.20, T42.3X2A
d. F13.20, T42.3X2A

84. The patient, a recent traveler from Hong Kong, presented with coughs, chills and high fever. The ER doctor wrote "SARS associated coronavirus" in the patient's chart.

a. Z20.89
b. B97.21
c. J12.81
d. B97.21, Z20.89

85. Code for malignant hypertensive nephropathy with uremia.

a. I12.9, N18.2
b. I12.0, N18.1
c. I12.9, N18.9
d. N19, K65.4

86. Code for aortic valve stenosis with coronary artery disease associated with congestive heart failure; in addition, the patient has diabetes and massive obesity.

a. I06.1, I25.9, I50.9
b. E11.9, I35.1, I25.10, I50.9, E66.01
c. E10.9, I35.2, I25.9, I50.9
d. E11.9, I08.0, E66.9, Q23.0, I25.10, I50.9

87. Code for pathological plica, right knee.

a. M67.51
b. M24.369
c. M67.50
d. M24.369, M67.50

88. Code for left hand nail remnant after traumatic left thumb injury. The hand was caught in a sliding door at home.

a. S67.02XS, Y92.019
b. L60.8, W23.0XXA, S67.02XS, Y92.019
c. L60.8, S67.02XS, Y92.099
d. L60.3, S67.02XS, Y92.019

89. Asymptomatic, non-sustained, ventricular tachycardia, there are no prolonged pauses, predominant rhythm is atrial fibrillation with well-controlled ventricular rate.

a. I48.92, I42.8
b. I48.91, I42.8
c. I49.01, I42.8
d. I42.8, I48.91

90. Code for a follow-up exam to radiotherapy, dwarfism (NEC), and a personal history of myeloid leukemia.

a. Z08, Z85.6, R62.52
b. Z08, Z85.6, E34.3
c. Z08, E34.3
d. Z09, Z85.6, Q77.1

Payment Methodologies - 20 Questions

91. CMS has delineated three mechanisms for payment of medical and surgical procedures (inpatient vs outpatient):

a. ED Services (Emergency Department), Inpatient Surgical Services (DRG reimbursed), Freestanding ASC (Fee-based).

b. Outpatient Surgical Services (APC reimbursed procedures not on the "inpatient only" list), Inpatient Surgical Services (DRG reimbursed), Freestanding ASC (Fee-based).

c. Outpatient Surgical Services, Inpatient Surgical Services, Lab and X-Rays (Technical Component).

d. APC reimbursed procedures on the "inpatient only" list, Inpatient Surgical Services (ASC reimbursed), Freestanding ASC (Fee-based).

92. Acute comorbid, chronic comorbid, and comorbid reoccurrence refers to:

a. Medicare Part A condition codes
b. Medicare Part B condition codes
c. Medicare Part C condition codes
d. Medicare Part D condition codes

93. What is IPPS and what does it mean?

a. Known as the Inpatient Prospective Payment System.
b. Under the IPPS, each case is categorized into a diagnosis-related group (DRG).
c. Both answers are correct.
d. None of the answers are correct

94. _____ is one of the variables affecting DRG assignment.

a. Sex
b. Specialties (cardiology, orthopedics)
c. Race
d. Age

95. Report condition code _____ for non-diagnostic services unrelated to inpatient stay.

a. 25
b. 32
c. 51
d. 52

96. Which scenario below would indicate Medicare as the secondary payor?

a. The patient has ESRD and his Group Health Plan (GHP) coverage was the primary plan prior to the individual becoming eligible and entitled to Medicare based on ESRD in the first 30 months of Medicare eligibility or entitlement.

b. Has ESRD and GHP coverage after 30 months of Medicare eligibility or entitlement.

c. Has ESRD and COBRA coverage after 30 months of Medicare eligibility or entitlement.

d. Medicare is always Primary.

97. Medicare Part-D:

a. The annual deductible can't be more than $400 (in 2017).
b. The plan must cover at least two drugs in each drug class.
c. Plans must have a network of pharmacies that provide convenient
    access.
d. All of the answers are correct.

98. The main difference between modifier -80 and modifier -81 is:

a. The board certification of the assistant surgeon.
b. Amount of time the assistant surgeon spends in the OR.
c. Mod-81 is used to indicate the primary surgeon and Mod-80 is for the
    assistant.
d. Mod-80 is used for the primary surgeon, Mod-81 for the assistant.

99. What would you expect to happen if you submit a claim, on the UB-04,
for an observation service that spans more than two days?

a. The claim will be rejected by the intermediary and returned.
b. This claim should be paid by the intermediary.
c. This claim would be paid if submitted on the CMS-1500 form.
d. This claim would be paid if Modifier -SG is appended to the observation
    code.

100. Can one use inpatient revenue codes to crosswalk to the correct APC
Code?

a. No, there is no tool for determining the APC by Revenue Code.
b. Addendum B provides the APC number by HCPCS Code
c. Both answers are correct.
d. Neither answer is correct.

101. Which of the below are/ is included on the charge description master (CDM).

a. DRG Codes
b. ICD-10 Procedural Codes
c. Both of the answers are correct.
d. None of the answers are correct.

102. There are nine ASC payment groups. Surgeries within a group are:

a. All paid the same amount.
b. All paid the same amount except for geographic differences.
c. Paid according to the specific APC code used.
d. Paid according to a formula derived from the ICD-10 diagnosis and the ICD-10 procedural Code.

103. The Hospital-based ASC must :

a. Be financially independent from the hospital.
b. Have its own Tax ID.
c. Not be on the hospital's cost report.
d. All of the answers are correct

104. The Outpatient Prospective Payment System is the same as the Inpatient PPS except that:

a. Fees for Inpatient procedures are higher.
b. The OPPS is based on the procedure codes, while the Inpatient PPS
      (DRG's) are based on the Primary Diagnosis.
c. OPPs allows for geographic differences.
d. There are no differences.

105. APCS are _____ than MS-DRGS.

a. The same
b. Different
c. More numerous
d. Less numerous

106. Payment status codes G and H are:

a. "Pass through" codes which allow additional reimbursement.
b. Inpatient Services that are not reimbursed under OPPS.
c. Outlier and Ancillary Codes.
d. Codes that are exempt from the multiple procedure payment reduction.

107. The multiple procedure payment reduction:

a. Applies when both surgeries and diagnostic procedures are performed during the same operative session.
b. Applies only to surgical procedures.
c. Applies only to cardiology procedures.
d. Applies only to codes with a status indicate of "S"

108. Is it preferable to "bundle" all services and bill under the appropriate APC?

a. Yes, it is.
b. Yes, but on for surgical procedures.
c. NO, bills should be itemized and the fiscal intermediary system will package services automatically. Providers should report accurate HCPCS codes and modifiers to ensure proper payment.
d. There is not enough information to answer this question.

109. Since supplies and drugs are packed into the APC:

a. They should only be billed on the CMS-1500 form.
b. They should only be billed on the CMS-04 Form.
c. They should still be billed on the UB-04 as covered and not shown as
    non-covered services (for statistical purposes).
d. It is not necessary to show them on the claim form.

110. The following items on the ASC Approval List: sterile supplies, intraocular lens, anesthesia, emergency department, simple laboratory tests are:

a. All separately reimbursable under OPPS.
b. All bundled in the surgery reimbursement.
c. Reimbursed on a sliding scale basis: 100% for the first item, 50% for the
    second, 25% for the third, fourth etc.
d. Neither separately reimbursed nor bundled. These are all billed on the
    CMS-1500 form.

HCPCS Level II Coding - 40 Questions

111. DIAGNOSIS: Bilateral upper lid ptosis, by levator dehiscence.

ANESTHESIA: Local standby.

OPERATION: Repair of ptosis, by repair of levator dehiscence, bilateral upper lids.

PROCEDURE: The patient was taken to the operating room and placed on the table in the supine position. Cardiac monitor and IV were established by anesthesia, who administered anesthesia standby. The patient was prepped and draped in the usual sterile fashion for oculoplastic surgery. Tetracaine ophthalmic drops were instilled into the eyes. Attention was directed to the upper lids where very little skin fold was noted, consistent with her levator dehiscence. At 12 mm above the lash line, a skin mark was made across the lid in a gentle arch. This was performed on both upper lids and noted to be symmetrical. Lidocaine 2% with epinephrine was injected into the right upper lid along the skin-mark line, and the skin incision was made with a #15 blade. Dissection was carried down to the subcutaneous and orbicularis muscle, down to the orbital septum which was then opened superiorly, and orbital fat was encountered. With gentle dissection, the levator aponeurosis was noted. The dissection was carried to the tarsal plate and the anterior tarsal plate was cleared. A 5-0 nylon suture was used to re-approximate the edge of the levator aponeurosis back to the tarsal plate, thereby elevating the lid, until the lid position was approximately 1 mm above the limbus. A second and third suture was placed, one medially and one laterally, with good arch of the lid.

Attention was then directed to the left upper lid where the exact, same procedure was done, after anesthetic was injected. Again, dissection through the skin and subcutaneous and orbicularis muscle down to the orbital septum, which was then incised. Orbital fat was encountered, and the levator aponeurosis was noted. The tarsal plate was cleared from the orbicularis muscle, and again three sutures were used to reapproximate the levator aponeurosis back to the tarsal plate. With a gentle arch to the lid, the lid now elevated about 1 mm above the limbus. Since this was symmetrical, all suture knots were then secured permanently. The skin was closed with interrupted 6-0 silk sutures.

a. 67906-50
b. 67904-50
c. 67903-50
d. 67902-50

112. PROCEDURE: Sigmoidoscopy.

INDICATIONS: Performed for evaluation of anemia, gastrointestinal Bleeding.

MEDICATIONS: Fentanyl (Sublazine) .1 mg IV Versed (midazolam) 1 mg IV

BIOPSIES: No BRUSHINGS: No

PROCEDURE: A history and physical examination were performed. The procedure, indications, potential complications (bleeding, perforation, infection, adverse medication reaction), and alternative available were explained to the patient who appeared to understand and indicated this.

After placing the patient in the left lateral decubitus position, the sigmoidoscope was inserted into the rectum and under direct visualization advanced to 25 cm. Careful inspection was made as the sigmoidoscope was withdrawn.

FINDINGS: Was unable to pass scope beyond 25 cm because of stricture vs very short bends secondary to multiple previous surgeries. Retroflexed examination of the rectum revealed small hemorrhoids. External hemorrhoids were found. Other than the findings noted above, the visualized colonic segments were normal.

IMPRESSION: Internal hemorrhoids. External hemorrhoids Unable to pass scope beyond 25 cm due either to stricture or very sharp bend secondary to multiple surgeries. Unsuccessful Sigmoidoscopy. Otherwise Normal Sigmoidoscopy to 25 cm. External hemorrhoids were found.

a. 45330
b. 45330-52
c. 45330-22
d. 45331

113. INDICATIONS: Iron deficiency anemia with low iron saturation. Positive fecal occult blood test per digital rectal exam.

FINDINGS: DIVERTICULOSIS: Sigmoid Colon, not bleeding; few small diverticulum POLYP: Sigmoid Colon, 5 mm, 45 cm from anus, pedunculated.

PROCEDURE: Snare with cautery, Polyp removed; polyp retrieved. Polyp sent to pathology.

HEMORRHOIDS: Internal, Size: Medium.

DISPOSITION: After procedure, patient sent to recovery. After recovery, patient sent back to hospital ward.

a. 45330, 45333
b. 45333
c. 45338
d. 45330, 45338

114. DIAGNOSIS: Abnormal uterine bleeding.

PROCEDURE: The patient was transferred to the operating room where she was placed on the operating table, and underwent induction of general anesthesia in the usual technique without difficulty. She was placed in the vaginal surgery stirrups and examined. She was found to have a midposition, normal uterus, and benign adnexa. She was prepped and draped in the usual fashion for the operation. The cervix was grasped with a single-tooth tenaculum. The cervix was progressively dilated to admit the hysteroscope. The uterine cavity was sounded to 2 3/4 inches.

The hysteroscope was introduced. The endometrial cavity was noted to have some irregular thickening along the posterior uterine wall, consistent with hyperplasia. This was also consistent with the office biopsy taken preoperatively. No polyp formation was seen definitively. The endometrium was thoroughly curetted and submitted to pathology. The patient was awakened from anesthesia and transferred to the recovery room in satisfactory status.

a. 58558
b. 58561
c. 58562
d. 58563

115. DIAGNOSIS: Scar of the left mandibular line times two.

HISTORY: This patient has two scars from an attack last year that has left on her left jaw line with "dog-ears" on either end, and she desires revision of these areas for more normal anatomic reconstruction site. She, therefore, presents today for definitive revision of these scars.

PROCEDURE: With the patient in the supine position under intravenous sedation, 1% lidocaine with 1:100,000 epinephrine buffered with sodium bicarbonate was injected into the two scars in question along the left jaw line. Each scar measured approximately 1.5 cm in length. Having waited 10 minutes for vasoconstriction to occur, each scar was excised under loupe magnification with a #15 Bard-Parker. Hemostasis was obtained with the Bovie. The closure was performed with two layers of 5-0 Vicryl, followed by running, fine, 6-0 black nylon, again under loupe magnification. The patient tolerated the procedure well. Sponge and needle counts were reported as correct times two. She was brought to the recovery room in stable condition.

a. 11442
b. 11442 X 2
c. 12031-51
d. 12031, 11000-51

116. DIAGNOSIS: 1. Primary adenocarcinoma descending colon 2. Hydronephrosis, bilateral.

OPERATION: 1. Cystoscopy 2. Bilateral insertion of Double J stents.

FINDINGS AT OPERATION: Endoscopic examination of the urinary bladder showed no significant abnormalities. Double-J stent insertion as accomplished bilaterally with minimal difficulty in the patient's left side.

PROCEDURE: With the patient in the lithotomy position and under satisfactory general anesthesia, the genitalia were prepped and draped in a routine sterile manner. The McCarthy panendoscope was inserted, and 24-cm, 6-French, silastic, Double J stents inserted bilaterally with ease. The patient was then sent to the recovery room in satisfactory condition.

a. 52332
b. 52332, 50575
c. 50947
d. 52332, 52332-51, 50575

117. DIAGNOSES: 1. Chronic left anterior and posterior ethmoiditis. 2. Chronic left maxillary sinusitis. 3. Left middle turbinate concha bullosa. 4. Chronic right anterior and posterior ethmoiditis. 5. Chronic right maxillary sinusitis. 6. Internal nasal deformity causing nasal obstruction secondary to septal deviation.

OPERATION: Bilateral endoscopic sinus surgery including: 1. Left anterior and posterior ethmoidectomy. 2. Left maxillary antrostomy. 3. Left middle turbinate concha bullosa excision. 4. Right anterior and posterior ethmoidectomy. 5. Right maxillary antrostomy. 6. Septoplasty.

PROCEDURE: The patient was taken to the operating room and placed in the supine position. After adequate endotracheal anesthesia was obtained, the skin was prepped and draped in a sterile fashion. Lidocaine 1% with 1:100,000 epinephrine was injected into the region of anterior portion of the nasal septum; approximately 10 cc total was used. Next, a standard hemitransfixion incision was made, and a mucoperichondrial flap was carefully elevated. The junction between the cartilaginous and bony septum was separated with a Freer elevator, and the bony deflection, which was quite prominent to the right side, was removed using open-biting Jansen-Middleton forceps. The cartilaginous deflection was corrected by freeing up the inferior attachments of the cartilaginous septum, correcting the deflected portion of the maxillary crest, and placing the cartilaginous septum more in a midline position. The mucoperiosteal flaps were carefully replaced into their anatomic position and showed good nasal airway patency. The initial incision was closed using 5-0 chromic suture, followed by a plain gut suture to reapproximate the mucoperichondrial flaps. Reuter bivalve splints were then secured with a 4-0 nylon suture for stabilization effect.

Attention then was directed toward the left side, where a 0-degree endoscope was inserted into the left nasal passage. Lidocaine 1% with 1:100,000 epinephrine was injected into the region of the left middle turbinate and uncinate process. The left middle turbinate had a concha bullosa. This was obstructing the nasal passage quite significantly and the sinus drainage sites. This was initially removed using a Tru-Cut and angled-cut forceps to remove the lateral aspect of the left middle turbinate. Following this, there was much more improved air space, both medially and laterally.

The uncinate process was then removed superiorly to inferiorly with back-biting and side-biting forceps. The natural maxillary antrostomy was then visualized and was occluded with polypoid accumulation. These were cleared using the Richards Essential shaver, along with back-biting and side-biting forceps. The anterior and posterior ethmoid air cells were then entered and primarily dissected with the Richards Essential shaver, with the superior and lateral dissection carried out using a 30-degree scope and up-biting forceps. Upon completion of this, attention was directed toward the right side, where the same procedure was carried out with similar findings.

On the right side, 1% lidocaine with 1:100,000 epinephrine was injected in the region of the right middle turbinate and uncinate process; 10 cc was used. Next, the right middle turbinate was displaced medially, and the uncinate process was removed systematically, superiorly to inferiorly, with back-biting and side-biting forceps. The natural maxillary antrostomy was then removed. Findings showed marked mucosal irritation. This was cleared using a back-biting and side-biting forceps. The anterior and posterior ethmoid air cells were then entered and primarily dissected, followed by use of the 30-degree scope and up-biting forceps for the superior and lateral dissection. Extensive mucosal disease was noted throughout these air cells, also.

Following this, the dissection sites were thoroughly irrigated with normal saline, bilaterally. Gelfilm packing was placed in both dissection sites for hemostasis effect. The patient tolerated the procedure well and returned to the recovery room awake and in stable condition.

a. 31255-50, 31256-51, 31240-50-51, 30520
b. 31255-50, 31256-50-51, 31240-51-LT, 30520-51
c. 31255, 31256, 31240, 30520
d. 31255-50, 31256-50-51, 31240-51-LT, 30520-51

118. DIAGNOSES:

1. Left chronic anterior and posterior ethmoiditis.
2. Left chronic maxillary sinusitis with polyps.
3. Left inferior turbinate hypertrophy.
4. Right anterior and posterior chronic ethmoiditis.
5. Right chronic maxillary sinusitis with polyps.
6. Right chronic inferior turbinate hypertrophic.
7. Intranasal deformity causing nasal obstruction due to septal deviation.

OPERATION: Bilateral endoscopic sinus surgery, including left anterior and posterior ethmoidectomy, left maxillary antrostomy with polyp removal, left inferior partial turbinectomy, right anterior and posterior ethmoidectomy, right maxillary antrostomy and polyp removal, right partial inferior turbinectomy, and septoplasty.

HISTORY OF PRESENT ILLNESS: The patient is a 55-year-old female who has had chronic nasal obstruction secondary to nasal polyps and chronic sinusitis. She also has a septal deviation mid posterior to the left compromising greater than 70% of her nasal airway.

PROCEDURE: The patient was brought to the operating room and placed in the supine position. After adequate endotracheal anesthesia was obtained, the skin was prepped and draped in sterile fashion. Lidocaine 1% with 1:100,000 epinephrine was injected into the region of the anterior portion of the nasal septum. Approximately 10 cc total was used.

A #15 blade and the Freer elevator were used to help make a standard hemitransfixion incision. A mucoperichondrial flap was carefully elevated, and the junction with the cartilaginous bony septum was separated with the Freer elevator. The bony deflection was removed using Jansen-Middleton forceps. The cartilaginous deflection was created by freeing up the inferior attachments to the cartilaginous septum, placing it more on the midline maxillary crest. The initial incision was placed in its anatomical position and secured with a 4-0 nylon suture for stabilization effect.

Attention then was directed toward the left side. Lidocaine 1% with 1:100,000 epinephrine was injected in the region of the anterior portion of the left middle turbinate and uncinate process and polyps. Approximately 10 cc total was used. The polyps were removed using the Richards essential shaver to help identify the middle turbinate and uncinate process better. The uncinate process was removed systematically superiorly to inferiorly with back-biting forceps. Next, the maxillary antrostomy was identified and expanded with the back-biting forceps and showed polypoid accumulation in the mucosal disease on its opening site. The sinus linings were edematous but did not have any polyps in the inferior, lateral, or superior aspects.

The anterior and posterior ethmoid air cells were entered primarily and dissected with the Richards essential shaver followed by the use of a 30-degree endoscope and up-biting forceps for the superior and lateral dissection. Bright mucosal disease and small polypoid accumulations were noted through the sinuses also. The inferior turbinates had some polypoid changes on them also and showed marked mucosal irritation and hypertrophy. The mucosal polypoid accumulations were cleared using the Richards essential shaver. The turbinate was partially resected from mucosally but with good shape to it. It was not desirable to remove it in its entirety. Any obvious bleeding points along the edge were controlled with the suction Bovie apparatus.

The same procedure and findings were noted on the right side with 1% lidocaine with 1:100,000 epinephrine injected into the anterior portion of the right middle turbinate, polyps, and uncinate process; 10 cc total were used. The polyps were removed. The Richards essential shaver was used to allow better exposure of the uncinate process. The uncinate process was removed superiorly to inferiorly with back-biting side-biting forceps.

Next, a maxillary antrostomy was identified and expanded with the back-biting and side-biting forceps and showed all plate accumulations there also. The anterior and posterior ethmoid air cells were then entered primarily and dissected with Richards essential shaver followed by the use of the 30-degree scope and up-biting forceps for the superior and lateral resection. The inferior turbinates showed mucosal disease, polypoid accumulations, and changes. These were removed using the Richards essential shaver followed by a submucosal resection of the hypertrophied portion of the turbinate.

Any obvious bleeding points were controlled with the suction Bovie apparatus. A thorough irrigation was then carried out in the nasal cavity, and Gelfilm packing was used to coat the linings in the middle meatal regions. The patient tolerated the procedure well and returned to the recovery room in stable condition.

a. 31254-50, 31267-50-51, 30140-50-51, 30520-50-51
b. 31255-50, 31267-50-51, 30140-50-51, 30520-51
c. 31256-50, 31267-51, 30140-50-51, 30520-51
d. 30520, 31255-50-51, 31267-50-51

119. DIAGNOSIS: Lumbar radicular pain syndrome.

OPERATION: Selective root (nerve) sleeve injection on the left at L5-S1 with fluoroscopy.

PROCEDURE: The patient is taken to the block room, placed in the prone position on the x-ray table. Sterile prep and drape is applied. Local is with 3 cc of 1% plain lidocaine. Using fluoroscopic guidance, the neural foramen is obtained on the left at the L5-S1 level, confirmed with three views and the injection of contrast. The patient does note transient paresthesia on initial needle positioning, however, is not present on injection. Negative aspiration is followed with the injection of 0.5 cc of 1% plain lidocaine. This results in total resolution of the patient's pain complaint. She also notes some numbness in the left lower extremity which was in a similar location to that when it is experienced; however, this has not been continuously present. This is followed with repeat negative aspiration and the injection of 40 mg Depo-Medrol, 3 mg Celestone, 0.5 cc Wydase, and 0.5 cc of 0.5% ropivacaine. The needle is removed intact. There is no blood loss. There are no apparent complications. The patient is without complaints.

a. 64483, 77003
b. 64483, 77003-26
c. 64483, 72100 and 77003-25
d. 64483

120. DIAGNOSIS: Left cervical radiculopathy at C5, C6.

OPERATION: Left C5-6 hemilaminotomy and foraminotomy with medial facetectomy for microscopic decompression of nerve root. After informed consent was obtained from the patient, he was taken to the OR. After general anesthesia had been induced, Ted hose stockings and pneumatic compression stockings were placed on the patient and a Foley catheter was also inserted. At this point, the patient's was placed in three-point fixation with a Mayfield head holder and then the patient was placed on the operating table in a prone position. The patient's posterior cervical area was then prepped and draped in the usual sterile fashion. At this time the patient's incision site was infiltrated with 1 percent Lidocaine with epinephrine. A scalpel was used to make an approximate 3 cm skin incision cephalad to the prominent C7 spinous processes, which could be palpated. After dissection down to a spinous process using Bovie cautery, a clamp was placed on this spinous processes and cross table lateral x-ray was taken. This showed the spinous process to be at the C4 level. Therefore, further soft tissue dissection was carried out caudally to this level after the next spinous processes presumed to be C5 was identified. After the muscle was dissected off the lamina laterally on the left side, self retaining retractors were placed and after hemostasis was achieved, a Penfield probe was placed in the interspace presumed to be C5-6 and another cross table lateral x-ray of the C spine was taken. This film confirmed our position at C5-6 and therefore the operating microscope was brought onto the field at this time. At the time the Kerrison rongeur was used to perform a hemilaminotomy by starting with the inferior margin of the superior lamina. The superior margin of the inferior lamina of C6 was also taken with the Kerrison rongeur after the ligaments had been freed by using a Woodson probe. This was then extended laterally to perform a medial facetectomy also using the Kerrison rongeur. However, progress was limited because of thickness of the bone. Therefore at this time the Midas-Rex drill, the AM8 bit was brought onto the field and this was used to thin out the bone around our laminotomy and medial facetectomy area. After the bone had been thinned out, further bone was removed using the Kerrison rongeur. At this point the nerve root was visually inspected and observed to be decompressed. However, there was a layer of fibrous tissue overlying the exiting nerve root which was removed by placing a Woodson resector in a plane between the fibrous sheath and the nerve root and incising it with a 15 blade. Hemostasis was then achieved by using Gelfoam as well as bipolar electrocautery. After hemostasis was achieved, the surgical site was copiously irrigated with Bacitracin. Closure was initiated by closing the muscle layer and the fascial layer with 0 Vicryl stitches. The subcutaneous layer was then reapproximated using 000 Dexon. The skin was reapproximated using a running 000 nylon. Sterile dressings were applied. The patient was then extubated in the OR and transferred to the Recovery room in stable condition.

a. 63020
b. 63020, 69990
c. 63015
d. 63015, 69990

121. DIAGNOSES: 1. Hydrocele, right. 2. Epididymitis, right, chronic.

OPERATION: 1. Scrotal exploration. 2. Epididymectomy, right. 3. Hydrocelectomy, right.

FINDINGS: Examination prior to, as well as at this procedure revealed the presence of enlargement of the right epididymis with associated hydrocele containing approximately 120 cc of straw-colored fluid.

PROCEDURE: With the patient in the supine position and under satisfactory general anesthesia, the genitalia were prepped and draped in a routine sterile manner. A vertical incision was made in the right hemiscrotum, and the testicle and associated tunic delivered into the wound. Utilizing careful sharp and blunt dissection, the hydrocele sac was opened, aspirated, and dissected, as was the epididymis. The vas deferens was transected and ligated in the procedure. The patient's hemiscrotum was then drained with a small Penrose drain placed in a dependent position, followed by serial closure with 3-0 Vicryl. Sterile compressive dressing was applied. Blood loss was negligible. The patient was sent to the recovery room in satisfactory condition.

a. 54861-52-RT, 55110-51, 55040-RT-51
b. 54860-RT, 55110-50-51, 55040-RT-51
c. 54860-RT, 55110-51, 55040-RT-51
d. 54860-RT, 55110, 55040-RT

122. DIAGNOSIS: Bladder outlet obstruction.

OPERATION: Cystoscopy with transurethral incision of the prostate and transurethral resection of the prostate.

INDICATIONS: This is a 61-year-old black male with a history of renal transplant. He had a history of bladder outlet obstruction symptoms prior to his transplant. He was in urinary retention and has been maintained on an indwelling Foley catheter.

DESCRIPTION OF PROCEDURE: The patient was taken to the Operating Room and placed supine on the operating table after undergoing spinal anesthesia without difficulty. He was placed in the dorsal lithotomy position and the area of his genitalia and perineum were prepped and draped in standard sterile fashion. The #21 French cystoscope with the 30-degree lens was then placed through the patient's urethra and into his bladder. It was noted upon entering his prostate that there was a minimal amount of prostatic tissue obstructing the neck. In the prostate the neo-ureterocystotomy was noted to be in the upper right side dome of the bladder. There was a stent present. The ureteral orifice was not patent. The left ureteral orifice was patent. There were no mucosal abnormalities seen in the bladder, however, there were several cellules. His bladder was trabeculated and there was a cellule. The cystoscope was withdrawn then and the bladder emptied. The Van Buren sounds were then used to calibrate the urethra to 28 French, then and #24 French resectoscope sheath was placed into the patient's bladder. The scope was placed thorough the sheath with a Collings knife attached. A transurethral incision of the prostate was then made, first on the patient's right side form just proximal to his right ureteral orifice to the level of the verumontanum. This was then repeated on the left side without difficulty. That accomplished and the resectoscope was removed and #24 French loop was then placed on the resectoscope and it was placed back into the bladder. The median lobe was then resected with very few bites taken. Then the patient's left lobe of the prostate was resected without difficulty. We then resected the patient's right lobe of the prostate. Aopproximately four grams of prostatic tissue were resected, the resectoscope was withdrawn and the Ellik was used to evacuate these chips from the bladder. The resectoscope sheath was withdrawn and a three way #22 French Foley catheter was placed into the bladder and started on continuous irrigation. The patient was taken out of the dorsal lithotomy position. He was then transferred to the stretcher and taken to the postoperative holding area in stable condition. There were no complications during the case, estimated blood loss was 50 cc.

a. 52601
b. 50948
c. 52402
d. 52601, 52402

123. DIAGNOSIS: Macromastia

ANESTHESIA: General

OPERATION: McKissock reduction mammoplasty, inferior pedicle only.

PROCEDURE: Under adequate general anesthesia, the breasts were prepped and draped in a routine fashion and injected with 0.5% Xylocaine with 1:200,000 epinephrine to aid in hemostasis. The patient's breasts had been marked for standard McKissock reduction mammoplasty preoperatively with the patient in the sitting position.

The right breast was operated upon first, and a standard McKissock reduction mammoplasty was carried out, creating medial and lateral flaps and excising medial and lateral triangles. The nipple was supported with an inferior pedicle approximately 10 cm. in width. Good viability of the nipple was present at the termination of dissection. Approximately 1,000 grams of breast tissue was removed from the left breast, and 1,000 grams from the right breast. The patient's wounds were closed with clear and black nylon fine sutures. Sterile dressings were applied, and the patient returned to the recovery room in satisfactory condition with a bra in place. Both breasts were operated upon in equal fashion. No drains were placed. There were no complications.

a. 19318
b. 19318-51
c. 19318-50
d. 19324

124. DIAGNOSIS: Dorsal ganglion cyst, left wrist.

OPERATION: Excision of dorsal ganglion cyst.

FINDINGS AT OPERATION: This patient had one of these thick, very firm cysts in the classic location beneath the extensor tendon.

PROCEDURE: The patient was given a general anesthetic, and the arm was prepped and draped in a sterile fashion, with a well-padded tourniquet around the arm. The tourniquet was inflated to 250 mmHg after exsanguination with an Esmarch bandage. A transverse incision was made over the cyst, carried down through subcutaneous tissue. The extensor retinaculum was incised, and tendons were protected with retractors. The cyst was then surrounded and lifted up off the carpus, taking a portion of the dorsal ligament. Irrigation was then carried out. The incision was closed with nylon and Steri-Strips. A sterile dressing was applied. The patient appeared to tolerate the procedure well.

a. 25111-LT
b. 25112-LT
c. 20612, 25111
d. 20612, 25112

125. Two benign tumors were removed via esophagoscopy, (rigid) via snare technique. Two additional benign tumors were removed via hot biopsy forceps. The correct CPT codes are:

a. 43216, 43217-51
b. 43216 X 2, 43217 X 2
c. 43216 X 2, 43217-51 X 2
d. 43216, 43217-52

126. DIAGNOSIS: 1. Hematuria. 2. Chronic Prostatitis. 3. Right ureteral stricture.

Operation: 1. Cystoscopy. 2. Bilateral Retrogrades. 3. Ureteroscopy.

HISTORY: Patient is a 69-year-old male with persistent microscopic hematuria.

PROCEDURE: After satisfactory general anesthesia was achieved, the patient was placed in the lithotomy position. A 21-French scope with a 30-degree lens was utilized. A survey of the bladder revealed some moderate hematuria and blood oozing from the enlarged median lobe of the prostate. The trigone area itself was elevated secondary to this enlargement.

The right ureteral orifice was cannulated with a #8 cone-tipped catheter, and a retrograde was performed. This revealed a small distal ureteral stricture. Otherwise, no abnormalities were noted. Similarly, a left retrograde was obtained. No abnormality was noted.

A ureteroscopy was performed to the level of the stricture on the right side using the #7 mini scope. This appeared to be a soft inflammatory stricture, as if there had been a small stone pass through there recently. Otherwise no abnormalities were noted. This was not balloon dilated. The bladder was drained, and he was awakened and transferred to recovery.

a. 52334, 74420
b. 52351, 74420
c. 52351, 74485
d. 52000 52005-51, 52351-51, 52334-51, 74420

127. DIAGNOSIS: Multiple Myeloma

OPERATION: Placement of P.A.S. Port, left arm

INDICATIONS: The patient, age 48, is currently under therapy for multiple myeloma and will require chronic venous access for continued treatment. She was referred for placement of a P.A.S. port device in the left arm.

PROCEDURE: This patient was placed on the operating room table in the supine position with appropriate warming and monitoring devices in place. The left arm was circumferentially prepped with Betadine and sterilely draped. 1% plain Xylocaine was used to infiltrate the tissue of the antecubitl fossa and good anesthesia was obtained. A transverse incision was fashioned through which a branch of the basilic vein was identified. A 5.6 French catheter and sensing wire assembly was inserted into the vein and its tip was advanced to the caval atrial junction. Catheter position was confirmed electromagnetically. The sensing wire was removed and the catheter was attached to a miniature port which was anchored in a subcutaneous space of the forearm.

a. 36556-LT
b. 36569-LT
c. 36561-LT
d. 36571-LT

128. DIAGNOSIS: Cataract, left eye.

ANESTHESIA: Topical

OPERATION: Phacoemulsification with intraocular lens implantation, left eye.

BRIEF HISTORY: This patient complains of progressive loss of vision and progressive cataract, admitted for phacoemulsification with implant. The patient is taken to surgery at this time for the above procedure. Technique is as follows.

PROCEDURE: The patient was prepped and draped in the usual sterile fashion. Following peribulbar and topical anesthesia with preservative-free lidocaine, a wire lid speculum was placed and the superotemporal conjunctiva was approached with a fornix-based conjunctival flap. A groove was placed 2 mm posterior to the limbus with a #64 Beaver blade and carried into clear cornea with an angled Beaver. A 3.0 keratome was used to enter the anterior chamber after a paracentesis was performed on the opposite side at the limbus. Viscoelastic was used to fill the anterior chamber and a capsulorrhexis was started in the center with a triangular flap, torn circularly in a counterclockwise fashion to complete a 360 degree anterior capsulorrhexis tear. Irrigation under the anterior capsule was then performed with Balanced Salt Solution to perform hydrodissection, separating the nucleus from peripheral cortical attachments, spinning the nucleus free. The nucleus was then bisected with the phacoemulsification tip and rotated.

These hemispheres were then sectioned into quadrants and splitting was performed with the cyclodialysis spatula, and the cannula for the viscoelastic. The aspiration was turned up on the phacoemulsification machine into position #2 with higher suction. The remaining nuclear quadrants were aspirated and phacoemulsification completed without difficulty. The irrigation and aspiration machine was then used to clean up the peripheral cortex and polish the posterior capsule. An 11 diopter lens was then rotated into position over the capsular bag. The inferior haptic was rotated into the bag and the superior haptic dialed into the bag. Miostat was used to constrict the pupil. The viscoelastic was removed under irrigation and aspiration control. One-half cc of Tobramycin and Decadron, 20 mg vancomycin were injected subconjunctivally at the end of the case. Maxitrol ointment and pressure patch were applied. The patient returned to the recovery room in good condition, to be discharged as an outpatient.

The patient will be submitted to optometrist, Henry Glenn for the full 90-days co-management. Forms have been completed and all necessary information has been sent to the optometrist. The patient knows that all follow-up care will be provided by Dr. Henry Glenn, OD.

a. 66982-LT
b. 66984-LT
c. 66984-LT-55
d. 66984-LT-54

129. DIAGNOSIS: Post dural puncture headache.

ANESTHESIA: Intravenous sedation

OPERATION: Epidural blood patch.

PROCEDURE: After satisfactory explanation of the risks and benefits of the procedure, patient was placed in the sitting position. His back was prepped with Betadine in a sterile fashion. A lidocaine skin wheal was made in approximately the L2-3 interspace. This site was approximately 2-3 cm above the superior aspect of a midline lumbar scar. A 17-gauge epidural needle was directed into the epidural space using loss-of-resistance-to-air technique. Negative aspiration for blood or cerebrospinal fluid was obtained. Twenty cc of blood was drawn sterilely from the right antecubital fossa. This was then injected slowly into the epidural space. Patient received 2 mg Versed during this procedure. He was taken to the recovery room in stable condition. He had good, though not complete resolution of his headache.

a. 62273
b. 62273-26
c. 62281
d. 62284

130. DIAGNOSIS: Right shoulder impingement syndrome, acromioclavicular joint arthritis, and rotator cuff tear.

ANESTHESIA: General.

PROCEDURE: Subacromial decompression and open rotator cuff repair.

In the preoperative holding area, the site, side, and procedure were confirmed with the patient. The risks, benefits, and alternatives were discussed and the patient voiced his desire to proceed. After adequate general anesthesia, the patient was carefully placed in the beach chair position. All bony areas were well padded. Careful attention was taken not to hyperflex the spine. After the shoulder was prepped and draped in a sterile fashion, anatomic landmarks were used to identify the portals. A posterior portal was established. The inside-out technique was used to establish an anterior portal.

The joint was inspected and found to have diffuse degenerative changes. Limited debridement was performed. The biceps tendon was absent. There was no evidence of a dislocation. The bald spot appeared to be normal. I think basically what we were seeing on the MRI was a bald spot with hypertrophic osteophyte.

Subacromial decompression was performed through the subacromial space using a burr. The acromioclavicular ligament was resected. A cutting block technique was used to make sure that adequate decompression was performed. Then a straight lateral approach was made for a mini-open repair of the rotator cuff which was repaired. The supraspinatus tendon and infraspinatus tendon were involved. Two suture anchors were used. Excellent fixation with water-tight closure was obtained with full range of motion achieved without remaining impingement.

The deltoid in the limited extent where it had been released was repaired back to bone. Multi-layered closure was performed. A Stryker pain pump was installed. A dressing was applied. The patient was aroused from anesthesia and taken to the recovery room in stable condition.

a. 29826, 23412
b. 29826, 23412-51
c. 23412
d. 23412-51

131. DIAGNOSES: 1. Sixty-percent degenerative left rotator cuff tear, joint side. 2. Impingement syndrome.

OPERATION: 1. Arthroscopic subacromial decompression. 2. Repair of rotator cuff through mini-arthrotomy.

FINDINGS AT OPERATION: The patient's glenohumeral joint was completely clear, other than obvious tear of the rotator cuff. The midportion of this appeared to be complete, but for the most part, this was about a 60% rupture of the tendon. This was confirmed later when the bursal side was opened up. note, the patient also had abrasion of the coracoacromial ligament under the anterolateral edge of the acromion. He did not have any acromioclavicular joint pain or acromioclavicular joint disease noted.

PROCEDURE: He was given an anesthetic, examined, prepped, and draped in a sterile fashion in a beach-chair position. The shoulder was instilled with fluid from posteriorly, followed by the arthroscope. The shoulder was instilled with fluid from posteriorly, followed by the arthroscope. Arthroscopy was then carried out in standard fashion using a 30-degree Dionic scope. With the scope in the posterior portal, the above findings were noted, and an anterior portal was established. A curved shaver was placed for debridement of the tear. I established this was about a 60-70% tear with a probable complete area of tear which was very small. There were no problems at the biceps or the rest of the joint. The subacromial space showed findings, as noted above, and a thorough subacromial decompression was carried out with a Bovie, rotary shaver, and bur. I did not debride the acromioclavicular joint. The lateral portal was then extended to a mini-arthrotomy, and subacromial space was entered by blunt dissection through the deltoid. The area of weakness of the tendon was found, and was transversely cut, and findings were confirmed.

The diseased tissue was removed, and the greater tuberosity was abraded with a rongeur. Tendon-to-tendon repair was then carried out with buried sutures of 2-0 Ethibond, giving a very nice repair. The shoulder was carried through a range of motion. I could see no evidence of impingement. Copious irrigation was carried out. The deltoid deep fascia was anatomically closed, as was the superficial fascia. The subcutaneous tissue and skin were closed in layers. A sterile dressing was applied. The patient appeared to tolerate the procedure well.

a. 29824, 23410-51
b. 29825, 23412-51
c. 29826, 23412-51
d. 29827, 23415-51

132. DIAGNOSIS: Foreign body, ball of left foot.

NAME OF OPERATION: Excision of foreign body, ball of left foot.

ANESTHESIA: General, tube balanced.

PROCEDURE: This 24-year-old lady was taken to surgery with the finding of a very tender isolated spot at the ball of the left foot between the first and second toes. By history, she felt like she stepped on something with pain, and over the ensuing week-and-a-half to two weeks the pain has gotten unbearable when she walks. X-rays did not show evidence of a foreign body. However, there is definitely a callous, granulous formation here that could possibly be a plantar wart.

In the operating room in the supine position after induction of adequate per Anesthesia, the left foot was prepped with Hibiclens and alcohol for a full three-minute prep. Drapes were applied exposing the ball of the foot only. Local infiltration of 0.5 cc of 2% Xylocaine was carried out. The area was elliptically excised, noting a very thick granular reaction beneath this. This was sent for permanent second. Total excision area was approximately 8 mm x 3 mm. There was no reaction deep to this.

With this, the wound was closed with two interrupted 5-0 Monocryl stitches giving complete closure. The area was cleansed with peroxide. A dressing was applied, and the patient was sent to the recovery room in satisfactory condition. Sponge count, needle count, and instrument counts were correct times three.

a. 10120
b. 11420
c. 28090
d. 28190

133. DIAGNOSIS: 1. Chronic cholecystitis. 2. Chronic cholelithiasis.

OPERATION: Laparoscopic cholecystectomy.

ANESTHESIA: General, tube balanced.

PROCEDURE: This healthy 42-year-old gentleman was taken to surgery with symptomatic gallbladder disease.

In the operating room in the supine position after induction of adequate general anesthesia without event, the anterior abdominal wall was prepped with Hibiclens and alcohol and shaved. Drapes were applied. A routine umbilical port cutdown was performed with direct visualization of the peritoneal cavity. A blunt trocar was inserted. Insufflation was carried out.

The abdominal contents were examined. There were no gross abnormalities. The gallbladder was tense and thick-walled, but there were no other findings in the pelvis or upper abdominal regions.

The remaining three trocars were inserted, and a routine laparoscopic cholecystectomy was performed, identifying the cystic duct, cystic artery, and the top of the common bile duct. Once said structures were identified, the cystic duct and artery were doubly clipped distally and singly proximally and divided. The gallbladder was dissected from the fossa in a retrograde fashion. The specimen was opened on the back table after it had been extracted through the epigastric port with removal of two large cholesterol stones. The mucosa was intact. The wall was definitely thickened with indications of chronic scarring.

Re-inspection of the gallbladder fossa showed excellent hemostasis. No bile leakage. The clips were intact. The area was irrigated and suctioned dry. This concluded the procedure. Routine abdominal wall midline closures were carried out. Band-aid dressings were applied, and the patient was sent to the recovery room in satisfactory condition. Sponge count, needle count, and instrument counts were correct times 3.

a. 47562
b. 47563
c. 47564
d. 47570

134. DIAGNOSIS: Left inguinal hernia.

ANESTHESIA: General; 0.25% Marcaine at trocar sites.

TITLE OF PROCEDURE: Laparoscopic left inguinal hernia repair.

A skin incision was placed at the umbilicus where the left rectus fascia was incised anteriorly. The rectus muscle was retracted laterally. Balloon dissector was passed below the muscle and above the peritoneum. Insufflation and deinsufflation were done with the balloon removed. The structural balloon was placed in the preperitoneal space and insufflated to 10 mmHg carbon dioxide. The other trocars were placed in the lower midline times two. The hernia sac was easily identified and was well defined. It was dissected off the cord anteromedially. It was an indirect sac. It was taken back down and reduced into the peritoneal cavity. Mesh was then tailored and placed overlying the defect, covering the femoral, indirect, and direct spaces, tacked into place. After this was completed, there was good hemostasis. The cord, structures, and vas were left intact. The trocars were removed. The wounds were closed with 0 Vicryl for the fascia, 4-0 for the skin. Steri-Strips were applied. The patient was awakened and carried to the recovery room in good condition, having tolerated the procedure well.

a. 49650
b. 49651
c. 49505
d. 49507

135. DIAGNOSIS: Conductive deafness, left ear.

Operation: Tympanoplasty with ossicular chain reconstruction.

PROCEDURE: Under general endotracheal plus 2% Xylocaine endaural block anesthesia, the ear was inspected. The patient had several surgical procedures performed on this ear over the years, the last one being approximately three months ago, at which time the tympanic membrane was totally reconstructed, and the ossicular chain reconstructed using an hydroxyapatite prosthesis from the stapes head to the underside of the cartilage-reinforced drumhead. At the time of this present operation, the drum head was intact and slightly lateralized. The middle ear was entered through a posterior tympanomeatal incision, and it was found that the hydroxyapatite prosthesis was lying free in the inferior part of the middle ear with the shaft still touching the stapes head, but the head attached to the medial wall of the middle ear.

This prosthesis was carefully dissected away. The medial aspect of the cartilage cap was scraped with a sharp right angle, and the reverse elevator, and then inspected with a Buckingham mirror to make certain that it was denuded of mucosa. Next, the middle ear was partly filled with moist Gelfoam. Another offset hydroxyapatite partial prosthesis was sculptured with diamond burs with approximately 0.5 mm extra length from the old prosthesis, with a groove cut for the stapedius tendon. This was placed in position with the chorda tympani touching this shaft at the medial aspect of the prosthesis. Using glue, the attachment with the stapedius tendon and the stapes head was glued in place. Then, the middle ear was completely filled with moist Gelfoam to stabilize the prosthesis. The chorda tympani was also glued to the superior portion of the shaft of the prosthesis. Next, the head of the prosthesis was covered with glue and the drumhead with the cartilage cap was replaced in position.

The tympanomeatal flap was secured in place with compressed, moist Gelfoam. External auditory canal was filled with Polysporin ointment. It was anticipated this ossicular reconstruction will stay in the proper position, and the patient will have a significant improvement in the hearing. The patient tolerated the procedure well.

a. 69632-LT
b. 69633-LT
c. 69635-LT
d. 69636-LT

136. DIAGNOSIS: Cardiac Tamponade

Ten-year-old boy was admitted with cardiac tamponade. Initial pericardiocentesis yielded pus.

PROCEDURE: A subxiphoid tube-pericardiostomy was done and thick, purulent material was drained out. Subsequently, pericardiectomy was undertaken as features of pericardial constriction persisted. At surgery, however, an intrapericardial mass was discovered. Successful excision was performed and the patient made an uneventful recovery. Histopathology of the mass revealed features of an intrapericardial teratoma.

a. 33015, 33020
b. 33015, 33020, 33050
c. 33015, 33050
d. 33020, 33050

137. Code for an EGD; with endoscopic mucosal resection.

a. 43251
b. 43252
c. 43253
d. 43254

138. Code for upper gastrointestinal endoscopy including esophagus, stomach, and duodenum with transendoscopic stent placement.

a. 43257
b. 43259
c. 43266
d. 43270

139. Code for transabdominal amnioinfusion using ultrasound guidance:

a. 59070
b. 59072, 76801
c. 59074, 76802
d. 59897, 76805

140. The surgeon performed arthrodesis of the vertebral bodies, L1, L2 and L3 (total of 3), using a lateral extracavitary approach of L1 (lumbar). A minimal discectomy was performed to prepare the interspace.

a. 22533
b. 22533-22
c. 22533 X 3
d. 22533 + 22534 X 2

141. The procedure was a vaginal colpopexy to reposition the patient's vagina . Approach was intra-peritoneal. During the procedure, the vagina was sutured to the sacrospinous ligament to secure it in place.

a. 57283, 57556
b. 57283, 58263, 58292
c. 57283, 58263
d. None of the answers are correct.

142. The surgeon performed an arthrodesis, including a laminectomy of the L1 and L2 segments. Approach was posterior with a posterior interbody technique.

a. 22630, 22632
b. 22633 X 2
c. 22634 X 2
d. 22633, 22634

143. PREOPERATIVE DIAGNOSIS: Right breast mass

OPERATION: Right subcutaneous mastectomy

INDICATIONS FOR SURGERY: Operative findings included benign-appearing breast tissue. Frozen section reports as benign breast tissue consistent with gynecomastia. The patient is a 51-year-old male who presented to the clinic complaining of swelling in his right breast under his nipple and areola. He complained that this area was tender and was concerned about possible cancer. The patient was scheduled for outpatient procedure, breast biopsy versus subcutaneous mastectomy.

PROCEDURE: After obtaining signed consent, the patient was taken to the operating room and placed in comfortable supine position. After placing all proper anesthesia monitoring devices, EKG, blood pressure and saturation monitors, the patient's right breast was prepped and draped in the usual sterile fashion. Once this was completed, 1% lidocaine was used to infiltrate the inferior aspect circumareolarly and a #15 blade was then used to make an incision circumareolar from 3 o'clock and 6 o'clock to 9 o'clock on the nipple and small extending incisions were created laterally and medially at 3 o'clock and 5 o'clock.

This incision was carried down through the skin and into the subcutaneous tissue. Skin flaps were then created using Metzenbaum scissors. Allis clamps were used to secure the mass and the mass was dissected out using electrocautery Bovie. After excision the mass, the lateral border of the mass was marked with long silk, the superior aspect of the mass was marked with a short stitch. This was then passed off to pathology for frozen section. Inspecting the wound, the wound was dry. It was irrigated copiously with normal saline. A 3-0 Vicryl was used to reapproximate the subcutaneous tissue to obliterate the dead space and a 4-0 Vicryl suture was used to reapproximate the skin edges using a Vicryl subcuticular stitch. Steri-strips were then applied over the wound. A sterile dressing was placed over the wound. The patient tolerated the procedure well and there were no complications. A total of 7 cc of 1% lidocaine were used during the case. The estimated blood loss was less than 10 cc. There were no drains.

a. 19302
b. 19302-RT
c. 19300
d. 19300-RT

144. DIAGNOSIS: Full-thickness nasal defect, skin of right alar.

ANESTHESIA: Local

OPERATION: Full-thickness skin graft of right preauricular area to right nose, 1 x 1 x 1 cm.

PROCEDURE: The patient had undergone Mohs' micrographic skin cancer surgery by another physician. I was asked to perform a skin graft to close the defect. She had an alar defect 1 x 1 x 1 cm, and this was fairly deep. She had previous basal cell carcinoma surgery just above that, preventing a nasolabial flap. The preauricular area was selected as site of the skin graft. This was marked and infiltrated with lidocaine with epinephrine, as was the nose. The preauricular skin graft was harvested in a hairless area just in front of the tragus, and the skin closed with 5-0 PDS and running 5-0 plain. Steri-Strips were applied. The skin graft was then defatted, trimmed to fit exactly into the defect and sutured into place with interrupted 5-0 plain and quilting sutures of 5-0 plain. The dressing was then applied. The patient was taken to the outpatient unit in satisfactory condition with stable vital signs.

a. 15260, 15004-51
b. 15260, 15002-51
c. 15260
d. 15004, 15261-51

145. DIAGNOSIS: right-sided trigeminal neuralgia refractory to medical care.

Microvascular decompression of the trigeminal nerve using the operating microscope suboccipital cranioplasty using methyl methacrylate and titanium mesh.

ANESTHESIA: general-endotracheal anesthesia

PROCEDURE: On call to the operating room, the patient received 1 gm of vancomycin intravenous Soluset. She was taken to the operating room where arterial and venous lines were placed by the anesthesiologist. General-endotracheal anesthesia was then performed. The patient was administered 80 mg of gentamicin intravenously. Foley catheter was placed under sterile condition. TED stockings and Venodyne boots were placed on the lower extremities.

The patient was then given 500 cc of 20% mannitol intravenous Soluset. She was placed on the operating room table in the supine position; a rolled towel was placed under the right shoulder. A Mayfield head clamp was fixated with 60-pound inches of pressure. The occipital pins were placed in the left occipital region and a frontal pin was placed over the lateral aspect of the right supraorbital ridge. With 60-pound inches of pressure, the head was fixated now into position, turned to the left, with the chin almost to the point of the left shoulder. The neck was noted to be supple. Slight flexion was performed, but it was possible to place two fingers underneath the chin at all times.

With the fixator in position, it was now possible to visualize the right suboccipital region. This area was shaved, prepped and draped in the usual sterile manner. The skin was infiltrated with a solution of 1% lidocaine and epinephrine.

The incision was now made extending from a point parallel to the upper aspect of the pinna, proximally to two fingerbreadths medial to the right mastoid, and extending inferiorly to the neck for a total length of approximately 14 cm. The incision was extended through the skin, subcutaneous tissues and through the muscular layers down to the periosteum superiorly. A subperiosteal dissection was performed using Bovie and periosteal elevator and cut down into the nuchal musculature. The self-retaining retractors were positioned. The entire suboccipital bone on the right side was thereby exposed, as was the mastoid bone.

Now the Elan-E drill was used with the perforator to make a bur hole in the suboccipital bone. Using a dental instrument and the Rhoton microsurgical dissectors, the dura was separated from the inner table of the skull. A sequential suboccipital craniectomy was performed using a combination of Leksell rongeur and Kerrison rongeur. The craniectomy was carried from approximately the lateral third of the cerebellum laterally to a point up to the sigmoid sinus. The craniectomy was carried superiorly to the transverse sinus and inferiorly almost to the floor of the posterior fossa. The dura was noted to be very tenuous through most of this area, and there were several durotomies in this segment as this was such thin tissue.

Once sufficient exposure had been accomplished at both the transverse and sigmoid sinus, incision was made into the dura and extended in a C-shaped fashion centered toward the asterion. A middle incising incision was carried straight toward this point and thereby two leaves were folded, one superiorly and one laterally.

Up to this point, the operative procedure had been carried using loupe magnification and fiberoptic headlamp. Now these were removed and the operating microscope was draped, brought into the field, and used for the remainder of the operative procedure. The dural leaves were tacked superiorly using 4-0 Surgilon sutures.

Using a hand-held retractor to support the cerebellum medially, it was possible now to identify the 7-8 complex and then progressing superiorly to identify the tentorium. Arachnoidal adhesions to the tentorium were bipolar coagulated and sharply divided. The dissection was carried posteriorly and the fifth nerve identified superior and anterior to the 7-8 complex. The petrosal vein was noted just superior to the fifth nerve.

Under high microscopic magnification, it was now possible to identify that there are two vessels in close approximation to the fifth nerve. One, a large branch of the superior cerebellar artery, was emerging from in front of the trigeminal nerve and coming superiorly. This was deforming the trigeminal nerve and pushing it dorsally. The second was a large vein that was running parallel to the inferior portion of the trigeminal nerve and was compressing it only slightly. The petrosal vein was not compressing the nerve at any point.

The dissection was carried along the nerve proximally to the root entry zone and the origin of the nerve in the pons. There was no pressure at this area, but only the artery and vein as described above, which were both located within 1-cm of entry of the nerve into the pons. Now using Rhoton microdissectors and micronerve hooks, it was possible to mobilize the arterial loop away from the nerve. It was noted that each time this was displaced back, once the vessel was let go, it would flip back beneath the nerve. It was, therefore, not possible to keep it freely away from the fifth nerve.

Now, Teflon felt was brought into the field and cut into very small wisps. This was now wedged between this arterial loop of the superior cerebellar artery and the trigeminal nerve. Several pieces were fashioned between these so as to completely separate the nerve from the artery.

Next attention was directed to the inferior portion of the nerve where it was noted to be in close approximation to the vein. Again, several pieces of Teflon felt were wedged between the artery and the vein thereby separating these two structures. There was no other point of significant vascular compression at any point along the nerve, which was examined in its entirety. The area was irrigated with saline, and there was no bleeding noted.

A piece of Gelfoam was now placed over the area of the incised dura, which could not be closed in a watertight fashion. The dural leaves were folded over and loosely reapproximated. The second layer of Gelfoam was placed exterior to the dura. Now the operating microscope was removed.

A cranioplasty was now performed in the following manner: A piece of titanium mesh was cut to the size and shape of the craniectomy and placed just under the craniectomy edges. The edges of the mastoid bone were copiously waxed with bone wax. Methyl methacrylate was prepared according to standard procedure, and as it hardened, it was placed into the craniectomy defect and molded and contoured so as to completely fill this area. As the acrylic hardened, it was copiously irrigated.

Now the self-retaining retractors were removed. The muscle layers were reapproximated with interrupted 2-0 Surgilon sutures. The fascia was reapproximated with closely-spaced interrupted 2-0 Surgilon sutures. A medium Hemovac drain had already been placed in a subgaleal plane and sutured to the skin. The subcutaneous layers were closed with buried interrupted 3-0 Vicryl sutures. Surgical staples were used to reapproximate the skin edges.

a. 61458, 62145-51
b. 61458, 69990, 62145
c. 61458, 69990-51, 62145-51
d. 61458, 69990, 62145-51

146. For revascularization therapy of the femoral/popliteal territory, how many codes should be used for a combination angioplasty, stent and angioplasty.

a. One
b. Three
c. One but use an Add-On Code for any additional vessels
d. None of the answers are correct

147. DIAGNOSIS: Recurrent right Bartholin gland abscess

OPERATION: Marsupialization of right Bartholin gland

PROCEDURE: With the patient in the lithotomy position under satisfactory general anesthesia, the perineum and vagina were prepped and draped in the usual manner.

The knife was used to incise an area of skin and exterior portion of the Bartholin gland, which was finished using Metzenbaum scissors. The specimen was sent for pathologic diagnosis. The lining of the gland was then sewn to the external part of the labia using a 3-0 Vicryl running locked suture.

Estimated blood loss was 25 cc. The patient tolerated the procedure and anesthesia well and was taken to the recovery area in good condition with no packs or drains in place.

a. 56440
b. 56441
c. 56441, 56441
d. 56440, 56441-51

148. DIAGNOSIS: Left knee medial meniscus tear.

OPERATION: Partial medial meniscectomy with limited debridement.

ANESTHESIA: General.

PROCEDURE: In the preoperative holding area the site and side and the procedure were confirmed with the patient. The risks, benefits, and alternatives were discussed. He voiced understanding regarding the limitations of arthroscopic treatment, particularly if there is arthritis involved.

The patient was taken to the operating room, and after adequate general anesthesia the left leg was carefully fitted with a tourniquet over a snugly-fitted Webril and placed in the left leg holder. The leg was prepped and draped in sterile fashion. Portals were carefully established using landmarks as a guide. The anterior-medial portal was established using a spinal needle as a guide. Sequential examination of the joint was performed.

Generalized arthritis was noted throughout except no full-thickness cartilaginous tears were noted. There was an unstable medial meniscus tear which was carefully debrided. The anterior cruciate ligament was a little bit incompetent with some fraying fibers, but no evidence of gross instability detected as pivot shift was equivocal. Hence this was left intact. The posterior cruciate ligament was normal. The patellofemoral joint tracked well. There were grade III articular changes throughout the knee. A few loose bodies were removed from some of the cartilaginous surfaces. The worst areas were smoothed, but otherwise it was left intact. Final inspection was made for loose bodies. These were removed. The last inspection found none.

The joint was irrigated and back-bled. The knee was injected with Xylocaine and Marcaine for pre- and postoperative pain. A sterile dressing was applied. The patient was aroused from anesthesia and taken to the recovery room in stable condition having tolerated the procedure well.

a. 27409
b. 29880-LT
c. 29881-LT
d. 29875, 29881-LT

149. DIAGNOSIS: Proliferative vitreal retinopathy, retinal detachment right eye. Status post trauma. Aphakia.

PROCEDURES: Scleral buckle revision, pars plana vitrectomy, membrane peeling, removal of silicone oil, PFO, fluid gas exchange, endolaser and reinjection of silicone oil right eye.

INDICATIONS: The patient is a 11-year-old boy who suffered a screwdriver injury to the right eye previously. He had undergone intersegment surgery by Dr. Smith for ant. Segm. reconstruction. Following this, he was noted to have a retinal detachment with a cataract approximately four months ago. At that time, he underwent pars plana lensectomy, vitrectomy, membrane peeling, endolaser, fluid gas exchange and injection of silicone oil with a scleral buckle to the right eye.

He was doing well until he developed recurrent proliferation superiorly with a superior detachment. He is taken to the operating room now for repair of the superior detachment.

PROCEDURE: general anesthesia. Using an ophthalmic endoscope a lid speculum was inserted straight in the right eye lid 2.5 mm inferotemporally a 5-0 Mersilene suture was passed in a mattress fashion and a 20 gauge sclerotomy created into the suture. A 4 mm infusion cannula space sclerotomy verified pin position inserted into place. Then the infusion was then turned on. The nasal sclerotomies were similarly created, a 2.5 mm posterior to the limbus. The superior detachment was noted to be anterior to the equator, between the equator and ora serrata superiorly. There were extensive preretinal fibrotic bands as well as subretinal fibrotic bands noted. The silicone oil was then removed form the eye. Following this, a Michel's pick was used to take off the preretinal proliferative membrane. The Dean forceps examination with the Michel's pick and vitrector were used.

The retrocorneal fibrotic band was present nasally from 12 o'clock towards 3 o'clock with a dense fibrovascular white band. Using a Michel's pick and vertical scissors the band was cut away from the corneal endothelium. Dewar pick forceps were used to peel off the fibrotic tissue. It was noted that there was a fibrotic band extending from the cornea onto the ciliary body and onto the retinal surface itself, which was responsible for tenting of the retina nasally. Following this, the view improved through the now more clear cornea in that location. There were still in the area of the corneal wound, fibrotic tissue which could not be removed. Following this, it was elected to pull up the scleral buckle.

Plugs were placed into the eye, the Wtazke sleeve and the ends of the 287 were identified superonasally. The ends of the 287 were trimmed an additional 3 mm. The Watzke sleeve was placed and the 240-band was tightened and trimmed. There was now a nice high buckling effect at 60 degrees. The plugs were removed from the eye.

The retinal tear was seen at 12 o'clock, which was felt to be the causative break. The previous break superotemporally still was attached and an additional laser reinforcement was placed to it. PFO was injected into the eye and all the subretinall fluid was drained out through the superior causative tear. Extensive endolaser was placed just around the tear superiorly as well as 360 degrees on the buckle. Following this the PRO was washed out with a fluid air exchange. Saline was injected into the eye. The sclerotomy superonasally was closed.

Silicone oil was injected into the eye for a good fill. Already present was an inferior peripheral iridotomy. The other sclerotomy was closed. The infusion cannula was cut and removed from that eye and that sclerotomy closed.

Five milliliters of 0.75% Marcaine was then injected using a blunt cannula into the retrobulbar space for postoperative analgesia. The conjunctiva was then closed. Ancef 150 mg and 4 mg of Decadron were given in a subconjunctival fashion.

a. 67107-RT, 67015-51-RT
b. 67108-RT, 67015-51-RT
c. 67108-RT, 66990
d. 67113-RT, 66990

150. INDICATIONS: Iron deficiency anemia with low iron saturation. Positive fecal occult blood test per digital rectal exam.

ANESTHESIA: Demerol & Versed.

PROCEDURE: Colonoscopy with polypectomy.

FINDINGS: DIVERTICULOSIS: Sigmoid Colon, not bleeding; few small diverticulum POLYP: Sigmoid Colon, 5 mm, 45 cm from Anus, pedunculated. Procedure: Bipolar Cautery, Polyp removed; polyp retrieved. Polyp sent to pathology.

HEMORRHOIDS: Internal, Size: Medium.

DISPOSITION: After procedure, patient sent to recovery. After recovery, patient sent back to hospital ward.

a. 45333
b. 45337
c. 45338
d. 45385

COC Mock Exam - Answers

Medical Terminology - 10 (Answers)

1. a. Surgical repair and ion of the boney components (bony contour) of the chin. Genio mean "chin". There is no genioglossus muscle.

2. c. Thoracotomy is an incision or cutting; -ostomy is creating an opening; - plasty is repair; - centesis is a puncture or perforation.

3. d. It is in the medial thigh region just above the knee.

4. c. Inferior occipital nerve. Vagus, Axillary and Pudendal are all valid somatic nerves. There is a greater occipital nerve, not an inferior occipital nerve. Since these are difficult to memorize, you can look these up in the CPT manual starting in the 64xxx range (although it may be prohibitively time-consuming).

5. a. A pneumothorax is a collapsed lung.

6. b. Enterocystoplasty: Repair of the bladder (bladder augmentation).

7. b. Surgical repair of a defect or wound in the urinary bladder.

8. c. Strangulated (hernia): An irreducible hernia that is trapped and cannot return to the abdomen. It is possible that blood flow can be cut off, gangrene can result and is considered a life threatening injury.

9. d. None. They both mean originating from within the body. These two (2) words are synonyms. -genic means "formed by", -logos means "relation". There is no difference.

10. c. Avulsion: Tearing away or forcible separation.

Anatomy - 10 Answers

11. c. Submental: Under the chin.

12. a. The ethmoid sinus is a honeycomb-like structure and is located between the eyes.

13. d. None of the answers are correct. Normally, you have two kidneys, one on either side of the spine under the lower ribs. They are pink in color and shaped like beans. Each kidney is about the size of your fist. The kidneys are two of the body' s most important organs. They are responsible for filtering the blood and eliminating waste products and excess water in the form of urine. Kidneys also help regulate blood pressure, make new red blood cells and maintain healthy bones. The body can function with one healthy kidney.

14. d. Frenulum: is a small frenula. There are numerous frenulum in the human body (e. g. , frenulum clitoridis, frenulum epiglottis, frenulum of prepuce (penis), frenulum of upper lip, etc. . .) The Frenulum of Morgagni is a fold, more evident in cadavers, running from the junction of the two commissures of the ileocaecal valve on either side along the inner wall of the caecocolic junction.

15. d. The medulla oblongata is the lowest portion of the brain stem, below the pons, as it enters the neck.

16. d. Pancreas. Endocrine portion secretes internally without ducts, but into the blood directly. The exocrine portion secretes outwardly to a free surface through ducts. The pancreas has both components.

17. b. The largest bone of the skull, superior to the occipital bone.

18. c. Popliteal area is beneath the knee.

19. c. In the Inner Thigh. The ADDuctor muscle is a muscle that draws a part TOWARD the median line. The ABDuctor muscle is a muscle that draws a part AWAY from the median line.

20. b. Atrial does not refer to a heart valve. The atrium is one of the heart chambers. The mitral is also known as the bicuspid.

Coding Guidelines - 6 Answers

21. d. 69620-RT. MYRINOPLASTY is the main term in the CPT index. Select code 69620. Removal of old tube, 69424, is not coded per the notes below the code. It cannot be used with codes 69433-69676. Only one code can be reported. One might argue that this is a separate procedure and submit 69424 with MOD-59 and the Operative Report for reimbursement.

22. a. FA-F9. Level II HCPCS to identify fingers are FA (left thumb) and then F1to F9 for the five fingers (including thumbs) on both hands.

23. c. Yes, but only on type "S" and type "T" procedures.

24. c. MOD-58 is used for staged procedures. Note that some insurance companies don't recognize and will not pay on this modifier. Skin grafts are often staged because you have to remove the skin from one area and move it to another.

25. c. Replace mod-59. There are four separate codes, each specific to the situation. Medicare introduced the codes in 2015.

26. b. Abuse. There is a difference between fraud and abuse. Fraud involves intentional deception or misrepresentation intended to result in an unauthorized benefit while abuse means charging for services that are not medically necessary, do not conform to professionally recognized standards, or are unfairly priced.

Compliance - 4 Answers

27. d. All of the answers are correct. To avoid interfering with an individual's access to quality health care or the efficient payment for such health care, the Privacy Rule permits a covered entity to use and disclose protected health information, with certain limits and protections, for treatment, payment, and health care operations activities.

28. c. Joint Commission on Accreditation of Healthcare Organizations (JCAHO) is a not-for-profit organization which operates fee-based, accreditation programs to subscriber hospitals and other health-care organizations.

29. c. All are valid components but the specific number is six. OIG is organized into six components through which we carry out our mission and support functions: the Office of Audit Services (OAS), Office of Evaluation and Inspections (OEI), Office of Investigations (OI), Office of Counsel to the Inspector General (OCIG), Office of Management and Policy (OMP), and Immediate Office of the Inspector General (IO).

30. a. While this is done, it is technically not allowed. This is a fundamental compliance concept.

CPT - 22 Answers

31. b. 27043-RT. Right hip, subcutaneous and soft tissue.

32. b. 57426 is correct.

33. d. 65820, Goniotomy; 66990-51. Use of ophthalmic endoscope (list separately in addition to code for primary procedure. Modifier -51 would be used because this is a multiple procedure. Get to know modifiers and when to use them. Code also the ophthalmic endoscope per CPT manual; this is a unilateral procedure, therefore MOD-50 is appropriate and MOD-51 for two procedures on the same day.

34. a. Use the New Patient Codes. Medicare stopped accepting E & M consultation codes several years ago. Use the new patient codes for Medicare patients. Check with each private carrier as some still accept the consultation codes.

35. a. 53210: urethrectomy, total, including cystostomy; female. Just one code, no modifier is necessary.

36. c. 45380: colonoscopy, flexible, proximal to splenic flexure; with biopsy single or multiple--one code, no modifiers necessary.

37. b. Morbidity refers to a disease or the incidence of disease within a population while mortality is the death rate as a result of a disease. Morbidity (mor-BID-eh-tee) (1) A disease or the incidence of disease within a population, e. g. , a morbidity study. (2) Adverse effects caused by a treatment.

38. d. When there is no presenting problem or chief complaint, then code the office visit as a preventive exam based on age. Codes 99381 - 99397.

39. d. 67550. An orbital implant is an implant OUTSIDE the muscular cone. 65130, an ocular implant is an implant INSIDE the muscular cone.
40. b. 50382: Renal Transplantation - Internal Dwelling Removal (Via Snare/capture) and Replacement of Internally Dwelling Ureteral Stent . . . via percutaneous approach.

41. b. Report 45171.

42. c. Include only those services performed by the discharging physician. The answer "Include all E & M services performed on the day of discharge could be ANY physician, therefore incorrect.

43. d. 52330: cystourethroscopy ; 52332-51: cystourethroscopy with insertion of stent. 74420: Urography, (pyelography) retrograde with or without KUB.

44. d. All the answers are correct. Coronary care unit, Intensive care unit, and Respiratory care unit. Highlight all the guidelines in the Critical Care section.

45. a. 52601 includes all the procedures listed in the question.

46. c. Add only same TYPE, same ANATOMICAL site grouping (per CPT codes). See the Guidelines in the Integumentary Section.

47. c. 16035-50: Escharotomy, initial incision. (removing eschar from a burn victim. 16036-50 X 2: Escharotomy, each additional excision. It requires bilateral modifier -50.

48. c. 43265, 43262-51. Look up ERCP in the CPT index. 43265: ERCP with endoscopic retrograde destruction, lithotripsy of stones. 43262-51: ERCP with sphincterotomy. MOD-51 means multiple procedures were used. Use on the second and subsequent procedures.

49. c. 33233: Removal of permanent pacemaker pulse generator only. 33212-51: Insertion of pacemaker pulse generator only; with existing single lead. Remember, code for removal and insertion. MOD-51 means multiple procedures used. Use on the second and subsequent procedures.

50. b. 37229. Key is with atherectomy (includes angioplasty within the same vessel).

51. b. J2150: Injection, mannitol, 25% in 50 ml. 100 ml was injected, twice the amount of the J code, therefore X 2 is correct.

52. a. G0127: trimming of dystrophic toenails, any number so one is correct. The S HCPCS code is not paid by Medicare and not accurate. Code 11719 is non-dystrophic.

HCPCS - 9 Answers

53. b. B9002. This is the correct answer because it states "any type" There is no code specifically for "with alarm." Without that it could be argued to use an unlisted HCPCS code.

54. d. J2360 x2, 90471 would be the correct answer. Myolin up to 60 mg either IV or IM. Since Myolin only goes up to 60 you would need to multiply the dosage x2 to achieve the correct dosage of 120 mg. 90471 is the correct administration code. The generic name is orphenadrine citrate.

55. b. Level II HCPCS Modifiers to identify toes are TA-T9. in the beginning of the CPT manual. P1 to P9 (anesthesia modifiers P1-P6) are incorrect on purpose.

56. b. J3240 X 2, 90471: The listed dosage is 0. 9mg. Therefore 2X 0.9 = 1.8 mg. 90471 is the correct injection code. 36415 is a venipuncture administration code, not an injection.

57. a. J1885 X 2, 96374. J1885 X 2 (dosage is per 15 mg) and the 96374 for the IV admin code. Multiply by 2 for the correct dosage. Ketoralac tromethamine is the generic name for the trade name Toradol; a nonsteroidal anti-inflammatory drug, is used to relieve moderately severe, acute pain. While this may seem difficult, an experienced coder should know some of the more common trade names to generic crosswalks.

58. c. Use MOD-33 for Medicare initial preventive physical exam (G0402) and AWV visits, G0438 and G0439. Do not use MOD-33 for services specifically identified as preventive: screening mammography, 77067; screening colonoscopy, G0105 or G0121; or prostate screening with PSA, G0103. The AWV has very specific Hx and documentation requirements (see Medicare website) and many common complaints (DM, HTN, OA) could be compliantly reported in addition with a level III code.

59. a. C1762. You can find this answer in the index of the HCPCS Level II manual by looking up the term Tissue, human origin.

60. c. HCPCS modifiers for the eyelids. E1 is the upper left eyelid, E2 is the lower left eyelid, E3 is the upper right eyelid, and E4 is the lower right eyelid. These are considered HCPCS anatomical modifiers.

ICD-10 - 30 Answers

61. d. Look up Wound, Open, Back in the index. Find S31.020A because it is considered complicated. Look up Accident, caused by a firearm, in the External Causes index. Find W34.010A, air gun also includes pellet gun. Confirm in the Tabular List. Look up backyard and confirm as location, the External Causes index. Find Y92.017 and confirm. ICD-10 codes: S31.020A, W34.010A, Y92.017.

62. c. G44.009: Cluster headache (more specific codes are available). R68.84 Jaw pain. M79.7 Fibromyalgia. F32.9: Depression NOS.

63. c. S06.333A, R56.1, V86.19XA. Fracture of vault of skull, loss of consciousness over 1 hour. Post traumatic seizures. Auto Accident, Passenger.

64. b. H92. 02: Otalgia, left ear (otalgia is ear pain that originates inside the ear). Z18.81: Retained glass fragments (means its been in the ear for awhile and no immediate plans to remove). This is less specific: H74.8X2: Other specified disorders of left middle ear and mastoid.

65. d. O80, Z37.0, assuming the this was a normal delivery without complications. The first two answers could not be correct because O80 is assigned only for a normal delivery w/o complications. Code O80 is always a principal diagnosis. O44.03: Placenta previa specified as without hemorrhage, third trimester (a condition in which the placenta partially or wholly blocks the neck of the uterus, thus interfering with normal delivery of a baby). This code would completely change the answer so D is the best answer.

66. c. D61.810 Antineoplastic chemotherapy induced pancytopenia. Pancytopenia is a reduction of one's red cell (anemia), neutrophil (neutropenia), and platelet (thrombocytopenia) count. A shortage in the amount of different kinds of blood cells, including: red blood cells, white blood cells, and platelets. Classic question construction requires clinical knowledge in several areas. Difficult.

67. c. J32.2, J32.0, J33.8, J34.3, J34.2. First main term is ETHMOIDITIS, code J32.2 Next main term is Sinusitis, subterm maxillary, code J32.0. Note that sinusitis, ethmoidal are also listed here. To code for the nasal polyps associated with the sinusitis, look under the main term, polyp, sub-term nasal or sinus, code J33.8 Hypertrophy is the next main term, sub-term turbinate, code J34.3. Deviated septum is the next term to look for, code J34.2. Five ICD-10 codes.

68. b. It means death or "to die". I21.3. Infarction is: The formation of an infarct, an area of tissue death, due to a local lack of oxygen. The obstruction of the blood supply to an organ or region of tissue, typically by a thrombus or embolus, causing local death of the tissue. The latin derivation means "to stuff or fill" but most think of it as cell death due to a blockage. Tricky question designed to make you think. Best answer is (b). I21. 3: ST elevation (STEMI) myocardial infarction of unspecified site [complete blockage].

69. c. H65.23, J35.03. The condition, otitis, is the main term in the ICD-10 tabular index for the first diagnosis. Chronic and serous are the sub-terms. Confirm the selection of H65.23 in the tabular list. Adenotonsillitis is a combined word. Break it down to two main terms, adenoiditis and tonsillitis. The coder finds the main term adenoiditis, sub-term chronic. Code J35.03 is selected because it is to be used for adenoiditis with chronic tonsillitis. Do not code separately for the hypertrophy. The notes tell the coder that hypertrophy is included in the code for adenoiditis and tonsillitis.

70. b. The foreign body is a ventilating tube placed by another physician. This is a retained foreign body. The coder looks at the main term, retained and is told to see retention. Under retention, there is a sub-term, foreign body, right middle ear, code H72. 91. To code the tympanic membrane perforation, the coder looks at the main term, perforation, sub-term is tympanum. Because the type of perforation is not specified, code H74. 8X1 is selected for right ear. Confirm ICD-10 Code H74. 8X1 in the tabular index.

71. a. S82.112B, W05.0XXA, Y92.019. A lot of specificity in orthopedics. Look up Home as the Location Y92. 019: Unspecified place in single-family (private) house as the place of occurrence of the external cause. Confirm in the Tabular List: S82.112B, W05.0XXA, Y92.019, S82.112B Displaced fracture of left tibial spine, initial encounter for open fracture type I or II.

72. c. G82.20, S24.2XXS. Look up PARAPLEGIA in the index. Note that this is a sequela of a previous laceration of spinal cord. You now must add the sequela code. Look up sequela and find spinal cord injury. The original spinal injury is not coded. The return visit is intentional, it's a test trick to misdirect.

73. d. None of the answers are correct. There are two main omissions. The cause and the ED codes are incorrect. There is no hypertension index in ICD-10. I15.1: Hypertension secondary to other renal disorders. The notes instruct the coder to report the underlying cause so you must include I77.3: Arterial fibromuscular dysplasia. N52.36: Erectile dysfunction following interstitial seed therapy. Z85.46: Personal history of malignant neoplasm of prostate.

74. d. R07.9, V43.51XA, Y92.410, Z04.1. R07.9: Chest pain, unspecified. V43.51XA: Car driver injured in collision with sport utility vehicle in traffic accident, initial encounter. Y92.410: Unspecified street and highway as the place of occurrence of the external cause. Z04.1 Encounter for examination and observation following transport accident.

75. d. S81.012A, key word laceration, knee. S61.411A, key word: laceration; right hand. W01.110A, Y92.099, Code location and instrument, 12032, 12004-51 code location and size adding together the wounds in the same location regardless how many. Remember that simple closure and single layer are considered the same type of closure.

76. b. R47.1, B94.1, Z51.89. Speech therapy converts to Z51.89, encounter for other specified aftercare code for dysarthria. R47.1, this should be reported as a sequela of viral encephalitis, note the word "following". B94.1 Sequela of viral encephalitis; note this is not an "S" type T sequela code.

77. b. H92.09: otogenic pain - of or originating within the ear, especially from inflammation of the ear. For H74.8x9 see Notes. Z18.81, retained glass fragments.

78. c. R31.9: Hematuria, unspecified. N41.1: Chronic Prostatitis. N13.5 Crossing vessel and stricture of ureter without hydronephrosis.

79. d. None of the answers are correct. Correct answers are: M84.463A (right fibula) and Q78.0 for osteogenesis imperfecta. Osteogenesis imperfecta indicates a pathological fracture. Fracture, pathological due to specified disease fibula, M84.46 and from the tabular M84.663 and the A is the appropriate 7th character for initial encounter for the fracture.

80. c. A40.9, B95.3. Look up SEPTICEMIA in the Index and find streptococcal A40.9: Streptococcal sepsis, unspecified
B95. 3: Streptococcus pneumoniae as the cause of diseases classified elsewhere.

81. b. T15.02XA, W31.1XXA, Y92.63. Note left eye is a two. T15.02XA: Foreign body in cornea, left eye, initial encounter. W31.1XXA: Contact with metalworking machines, initial encounter. Y92.63: Factory as the place of occurrence of the external cause.

82. a. K59.00, C81.99, Z85.72.

83. c. R40,20, T42.3X2A. Look up COMA, in the index. Confirm in the Tabular List. Since alcohol was involved, this is considered a poisoning. Code the Poisoning + Accidental Drug code + Alcoholic or Drug Intake. Do not code the ALCOHOL in Table of Drugs (Poisoning). Look up Seconal in Table of Drugs. Seconal: barbiturate that is a white odorless slightly bitter powder (trade name Seconal) used as a sodium salt for sedation and to treat convulsions.

84. b. B97.21. SARS-associated coronavirus as the cause of diseases classified elsewhere. There is no reference to pneumonia. If the patient has SARS, it could be argued that coding Z20.89, Contact with and (suspected) exposure to other communicable diseases, would be redundant.

85. c. I12.9, N18.9. I12.9 : Hypertensive chronic kidney disease with stage 1 through stage 4 chronic kidney disease, or unspecified chronic kidney disease. N18.9:Chronic kidney disease, unspecified. Uremia is a condition resulting from advanced stages of kidney failure in which urea and other nitrogen-containing wastes are found in the blood.

86. b. E11.9, I35.1, I25.10, I50.9, E66.01. Stenosis is the main term in ICD alpha index. Sub-term is aortic (valve). For the coronary artery disease, the main term is disease, sub-term coronary. When the coder confirms this code in the tabular index, it is noted that this is a nonspecific diagnosis. Coder then reads the description of diagnoses in the same section. This is a native artery (nothing in the description indicates otherwise). Failure is the next main term, modifying terms heart, congestive. Obesity is a main term, morbid is the sub-term. Diabetes is a main term. Select code because we have no information as to the type or manifestations.

87. a. M6751. To code the plica, look under main term, Plica, sub-term knee and then right = 1.

88. b. L60.8, W23.0, S67.02XS, Y92.019. Remnant is the main diagnostic term. Sub-term is nail. Confirm code in the Tabular List. Note that the definition of this code is: Other specified diseases of nail (an injury is not a disease) and X-walks to either L60.3 or L60.8. In the Index: Remnant fingernail L60.8, Crushing injury of finger. W23.0: sliding door and door frame. Y92. 019: Unspecified place in single-family (private) house as the place of occurrence of the external cause. S67.02XS Crushing injury of left thumb, sequela, L60.8 Other nail disorders not L60.9 Nail disorder, unspecified and not Q84.9 Remnant, fingernail is a congenital code, not L60.3 Nail dystrophy.

89. b. I48.91; unspecified atrial fibrillation, always code the reason for the encounter first. I42.8, other primary cardiomyopathies.

90. b. Z08, Z85.6, E34.3. Follow-up exam to radiotherapy a personal history of myeloid leukemia and dwarfism (NEC) and dwarfism. Z08, Encounter for follow-up examination after completed treatment for malignant neoplasm. Z85.6, Personal history of leukemia. [it appears the ICD-10 code is less specific; that does happen]. Look up dwarfism in the ICD-10 index and find 20 options; endocrine, pancreatic, renal, and congenital. But the GEMS cross walk is E34.3, Short stature due to endocrine disorder which covers several types. One could argue for the excludes code. Do not report with: short stature NOS (R62.52).

Payment Methodologies - 20 Answers

91. b. This is not an easy question. While it can appear to be overwhelming, (a), (c) and (d) have enough incorrect selections to allow selecting the correct answer by the process of elimination.

92. a. Medicare Part A condition codes.

93. c. IPPS for acute care inpatient hospital stays. Under Medicare Part-A (Hospital Insurance) is based on prospectively set rates, known as the Inpatient Prospective Payment System (IPPS). Under the IPPS, each case is categorized into a diagnosis-related group (DRG).

94. d. Age. The first three answers are not factors. Age is a factor.

95. c. Code 51 is correct.

96. a. Long list of scenarios on the Medicare as Secondary web page.

97. d. All of the answers are correct. The basic plan generally meets the following criteria:

The annual deductible can't be more than $400 (in 2017).
The plan must cover at least two drugs in each drug class.
The plan must cover substantially all drugs in these six categories: antidepressants, antipsychotics, anticonvulsants, antiretrovirals (AIDS treatments), anticancer drugs, and immunosuppressants.
Members must be able to seek an exception if a drug is medically necessary but not covered under the plan.
Plans must have a network of pharmacies that provide convenient access.
Lists of covered drugs and pharmacy networks must be readily available to members.
Plans must work with nursing homes.
Plans must help transition a member's current drug coverage.
Plans must offer catastrophic coverage that is at least as good as the coverage outlined in the 2003 Medicare Act.

98. b. Amount of time the assistant surgeon spends in the OR. Minimal means they both were there but it is not documented how much each contributed. Assistant means they contributed a significant amount of time to the procedure (but they are not co-surgeons, that's a different modifier).

99. a. The claim will be rejected by the intermediary and returned. Outpatient Observation services are intended to determine the need for inpatient admissions. Some cases may exceed a 24-hour period but observations services that exceed 48 hours will be denied as not reasonable and necessary. Also, observation cases may be converted to inpatient admissions, but inpatient admissions may not be converted retroactively to observation. Observation services are not appropriate for routine recovery from diagnostic testing and or outpatient surgery or procedures.

100. a. There are nine (9) categories of APC Code organized by complexity and the time involved for the surgical procedure. There is no crosswalk.

101. d. The Charge Description Master often contains the Department Number, an inventory control number, Revenue center code, CPT/HCPCS codes and a description of the service. DRG's are most often looked up using an Encoder (like 3M) and the ICD-10-PCS are either looked up in the ICD-10 manual or Cross-walked from the CPT Codes.

102. b. Nine groups. All APC's within a group are paid the same amount except for geographic differences.

103. d. ALL are necessary for the facility to be considered.

104. b. The OPPS is based on the procedure codes, while the Inpatient PPS (DRG's) are based on the Primary Diagnosis. This is a fundamental concept of inpatient versus outpatient facility coding.

105. b. Different. Outpatients can have multiple APCs for a given encounter, whereas an inpatient can have only one MS-DRG.

106. a. "Pass through" codes which allow additional reimbursement. G is for "Pass through" codes which allow additional reimbursement for current drugs or biologicals. H is for a device paid as a "pass-through".

107. b. Applies only to surgical procedures. Tricky Question. Status of "S" is for procedures EXEMPT from the multiple procedure reduction. Status indicator of "T" applies to significant procedure paid under OPPS (Outpatient Prospective Payment System), yet are subject to the multiple procedure discount.

108. c. NO, bills should be itemized and the fiscal intermediary system will package services automatically. Providers should report accurate HCPCS codes and modifiers to ensure proper payment.

109. c. They should still be billed on the UB-04 as covered and not be shown as non-covered services (for statistical purposes)" is the better answer.

110. b. All the items above are bundled in the surgery reimbursement.

HCPCS Level II Coding - 40 Answers

111. b. 67904-50. Main term in the CPT index is REPAIR. Modifying terms, are eyelid, ptosis, levator resection, codes 67903 –67904. Code 67904 is selected because the approach was external (on the outside of the eyelid). Modifier -50 indicates bilateral procedure.

112. b.45330-52. Sigmoidoscopy is the main term in the CPT index. The operative report does not indicate that the sigmoidoscopy was being performed for surgical reasons such as to remove a polyp or control bleeding. The coder selects the code for exploration, 45330. The operative report indicates that the scope was unable to pass beyond 25cm and states the sigmoidoscopy was unsuccessful. CPT guidelines state modifier -52 should be used when the procedure is not completed successfully.

113. c. 45338. The main term is the CPT index is Sigmoidoscopy, modifying terms are removal, polyp. Codes is 45338. Code 45338 is selected because the polyp was removed by snare technique.

114. d.58563. Coder should look under the main term Hysteroscopy, modifying term Ablation, then Endometrial.

115. b. 11442 x 2. Excision is the main term in the CPT index. Lesion, skin, benign are the modifying terms, codes 11400, 11471. The instructional notes in this section tell the coder that cictricial (scar) lesions are included. Code 11442 is selected because the site is face, and the size for each lesion is 1.5 cm.

116. a. 52332. Main term in the CPT index is Cystourethroscopy, modifying terms are Insertion, Indwelling Ureteral Stent. Code 52332 is selected. The description of this code gives double J stent as an example.

117. b. Ethmoidectomy, antrostomy, and septoplasty are the main terms in the CPT index. Excision of turbinate concha bullosa could not be found in the CPT index. This is a case where the coder has to read the sinus endoscopy section of the CPT manual until the correct code, 31240, is found. Modifier –50 is added to indicate procedures that were performed bilaterally. Modifier –51 is added to indicate multiple procedures.

CPT: 31255-50 31256-50-51 31240-51-LT 30520-51.

118. b. There are four procedures to code. All terms are found in the CPT index. First term is ethomoidectomy, endoscopic, codes 31254-31255. Select code 31255, ethomoidectomy, for total procedure. Add modifier -50 for bilateral procedure.

Second term is anstrostomy, maxillary, codes 31256-31267. Select code 31267 because polypoid material was removed. Add modifier -50 for bilateral procedure and Modifier -51 for multiple procedures.

Third term is turbinate, excision, codes 30130-30140. Note that these codes are for any method, which would include endoscopy. Code 30140 is selected because the body of the operative report indicates submucosal resection was performed. Add modifier -50 for bilateral procedure and modifier -51 for multiple procedures. Select CPT code 30520, Septoplasty. Add modifier -51 for multiple procedures.

CPT Codes: (4) 31255-50, 31267-50-51, 30140-50-51, 30520-51.

119. d. Main CPT term is INJECTION. Modifying term is nerve, anesthetic, code 64400 –64530. Code 64483 is selected because the approach was transforaminal (coder must obtain this information by reading body of report) and site is lumbosacral. CPT: 64483. To code for the fluoroscopic guidance, look under the main term, Fluoroscopy. Modifying terms are spine, guide catheter, code 77003. Do not code for 72100 -Radiologic examination, Spine, lumbosacral, two or three views - this will be billed by the facility. CPT: 64483 Do not code 77003-26 as this is included.

120. b. 63020, 69990. Hemilaminectomy and laminotomy mean removal of a portion of a vertebral lamina. The main CPT term is hemilaminectomy. Code range 63020-63044. Code 63020 is selected because the site is cervical and the code includes foraminotomy and facetectomy. Use code 69900 for the microscope.

121. c. 54860-RT, 55110-51, 55040-RT-51. Epididymectomy is the main term in the CPT index. Select 54860 because the procedure was unilateral. Modifier -RT is added to indicate right side. Exploration is a main term, modifying term scrotum, code 55110. (Modifier 50 would not be appropriate). Add modifier -51 for multiple procedures. Hydrocele is the main term in the CPT index. Modifying terms are unilateral, bunica vaginalis, code 55040. Modifier -RT is added to indicate right side and modifier -51 is added to indicate multiple procedures. Hydrocelectomy can also be found under the main term excision, modifying term hydrocele.

122. a.52601. The most direct way to find this procedure in the index is to look under the main term, Prostate, modifying terms Excision, Transurethral, which tells the coder to look at codes 52402 and 52601. Code 52601 is selection because a complete procedure was performed. The coder could also look under the main term Cystourethroscopy and read the description of each of the codes listed there to arrive at code 52601.

123. c. 19318-50. McKissock reduction: Marks the new nipple position with the blood supply of the nipple preserved on a pedicle of tissue the excess breast is removed. The nipple is then moved into its new position and the new breast shape reconstructed. The incision is often around the nipple and on the under surface of the breast, like an "upside down T".

Mammoplasty is the main term in the CPT index, modifying term is reduction, code 19318. Modifier -50 is added to indicate the procedure was bilateral.

124. a. 25111-LT. Excision is the main term in the CPT index. Modifying terms are ganglion cyst, wrist, codes 25111-25112. Code 25111 is selected because the operative report does not indicate this is a recurrent cyst. Add MOD-LT for the left wrist. note that the correct code can also be found under the main term, ganglion.

125. a. 43216, 43217-51. 43216: esophagoscopy, removal of tumor(s) by hot biopsy forceps. 43217-51: esophagoscopy, by snare technique, multiple Mod -51. Both codes include multiple lesions.

126. c. 52351, 74485. Ureteroscopy is the main term in the CPT index. Modifying term is with Cystourethroscopy. Code 52351 is selected because the ureteroscopy did not include other procedures such as biopsy or destruction. CPT instructs coders to use 74485 with 52351 for radiological supervision.

127. d. 36571-LT. Unless the coder knows what a PAS port is, he/ she should read the body of the report to determine that a catheter was inserted. Look under the main term Insertion. The age is greater than 5 years. This is a "non-tunneled" Insertion. There is a PORT. Code 3657 is selected because the patient is over five years of age, it is Non-tunneled, with a PORT. Add modifier LT for left arm.

128. c. 66984-55-LT. Phacoemulsification is the main term in the CPT index. Modifying term is extracapsular, codes 66982 and 66984. Code 66984 is selected because the report does not indicate a complex procedure. Modifier -LT indicates left eye. The coder must read the entire note to see that the surgeon is performing the surgical procedure only and all co-management (follow-up care) will be performed by an optometrist.

129. a. 62273. Main term in the CPT index is injection, modifying terms are spinal cord, blood, code 62273. This can be determined from reading the body of the operative report. The description of code 62273 confirms that is to be used for an epidural blood patch.

130. b. 29826, 23412-51. Code the Claviculectomy; partial 29826-51 Arthroscopy, shoulder, surgical; decompression of subacromial space with partial acromioplasty, with or without coracoacromial release. Code 23412: Repair of ruptured musculotendinous cuff, chronic. Add Modifier -51, multiple procedure modifier.

131. c. 29826, 23412-51. Both the arthroscopic and the open procedures should be coded. In the CPT index, first look under the main term, arthroscopy. Modifying terms are surgical, shoulder, code ranges 29819-29826. Code 29826 is selected because the procedure is decompression of the subacromial space. To code repair of the rotator cuff, look under the main term, rotator cuff, repair, which gives a range of codes, 23410-23412. Code 23412 is selected due to the chronic nature of the deformity. Modifier -51 is added to indicate multiple procedures.

132. d. 28190. Secondary Term is Foreign body, foot. Look up the code in the Tabular List. 28190: Removal of foreign body, foot; subcutaneous.

133. a. 47562. Cholecystectomy is the main term in the CPT index. A range of codes is given. Code 47562 is selected because the procedure was performed through a laparoscope. CPT: 47562: Laparoscopy, surgical; cholecystectomy.

134. a. 49650. The correct code for the hernia repair can be found two ways. Look under the main term, repair, modifying terms hernia, inguinal, initial, code 49650. Alternatively, look under the main term laparoscopy, modifying term hernia repair, initial, code 49650. This is considered an initial hernia because there is no information in the Op Report to indicate otherwise.

135. b. 69633-LT. Tympanoplasty is the MAIN term in the CPT index. The coder reads the operative report and determines that a prosthesis was inserted. The modifying terms in the index are with Ossicular Chain Reconstruction and Synthetic Prosthesis, code 69633. Modifier -LT is used to indicate the left ear.

136. c. 33015, 33050. A tube pericardiostomy was performed, therefore look up Pericardiostomy in the Index, 33015. Resection of pericardial cyst or tumor is 33050.

137. d. 43254. Esophagogastroduodenoscopy, flexible, transoral; with endoscopic mucosal resection.

138. c. 43266. Esophagogastroduodenoscopy, flexible, transoral; with placement of endoscopic stent (includes pre- and post-dilation and guide wire passage, when performed). An endoscopy of the esophagus, stomach, and duodenum is essentially the definition of an EGD, or Esophagogastroduodenoscopy. That is a little tricky but an example of how understanding medical terminology leads to accurate coding. 43259 does not mention stent placement.

139. a. 59070. This is a transabdominal amnioinfusion, which INCLUDES the ultrasound guidance.

140. d. 22532. thoracic, 22533 lumbar 22534 Add-On for either. Answer is 22533 + 22534 X 2 for three bodies. This is a difficult question.

141. d. None of the answers are correct. 57283 Colpopexy, vaginal; intra-peritoneal approach (uterosacral, levator myorrhaphy). See the list of codes that cannot be reported with this code in the CPT manual. Do not report the following codes: 57556, 58263, 58270, 58280, 58292, and 58294, with code 57283, since those codes already include enterocele repair.

142. d. 22633, 22634. 22633 Arthrodesis, combined posterior or posterolateral technique with posterior interbody technique including laminectomy and/or discectomy sufficient to prepare interspace (other than for decompression), single interspace and segment; lumbar. 22634 is the ADD-ON code for each additional interspace and segment.

143. d. 19300-RT. Main term in the CPT index is mastectomy and modifying term is gynecomastia, code 19300. Note this is a procedure on a male patient. Modifier -RT is used to indicate right breast.

144. a. 15260, 15004-51. SKIN is the main term in the CPT index. Modifying terms are grafts, free, codes 15002-15400. Code 15260 is selected because the graft was full thickness and site was nose. Code 15004 is used for preparation of the recipient site. Note that this is on the face.

Parenthetical notes tell the coder that the free graft and the preparation should be coded separately. Modifier-51 is added to indicate multiple procedures. The codes should be sequenced with the higher RVU code first.

145. d. 61458, 69990, 62145-51. Craniectomy is the main term in the CPT index. The modifying term, surgical provides the coder several codes to consider. Code 61458 is selected because the location is suboccipital and the nerve was decompressed.

The operating microscope was used and should be coded using code 69990, which is an add-on code and does not require the use of modifier – 51. Cranioplasty to repair the defect should be coded. The coder is given a range of codes. Codes 62145 is selected because the cranioplasty was to repair the defect at the time of the craniectomy. Modifier -51 is added to indicate multiple procedures.

146. a. One. The answer is found in the CPT Guidelines for this section which I highly recommend reading. Use a single interventional code, 37230, for the femoral/ popliteal territory and do not use Add-On.

147. a. 56440. Marsupialization is the main term, and Bartholin's Gland Cyst is the modifying term, which tells the coder to use code 56440.

148. c. 29881-LT. Name of operation does not specify that this was an arthroscopic procedure. [Note: these are actual op reports so spelling errors were left in]. Further reading of the report indicates that the procedure was performed through the scope (not an open procedure). Arthroscopy is the main term in the CPT index. Modifying terms are surgical, left knee, codes 29871 , 29889. Code 29881 is selected because only a medial menisectomy was performed. Limited debridement is included. Modifier -LT indicates left knee. CPT: 29881-LT.

CPT code 29881 identifies the excision of the disk(s) of fibrocartilage, called menisci, which divide some freely movable joints (either partially or completely) into two compartments located between the articular surfaces of the femur and tibia-one laterally and one medially.

Code 29875 would not be coded WITH code 29881. It would be considered bundled.

149. c. 67108-RT, 66990. This operative report is complicated and requires the coder to read it carefully to determine what procedures were performed and the associated diagnostic codes.

The coder looks up the main term Scleral Buckling in the CPT index, which says to see Retina, Repair, Detachment. This directs the coder to code: 67108. Note that the tear is 60 degrees (not 90 or more). The revised code now includes aspiration or drainage of fluid (formerly a separate code 67015). Modifier -51 is used to indicate multiple procedures.

150. a. 45333. The main term is the CPT index is Sigmoidoscopy, modifying terms are removal, polyp. Code 45333 is selected because the polyp was removed by bipolar cautery.

Left Blank Intentionally.

Scoring Sheets
Tear out for easy use

1)	A	B	C	D	29)	A	B	C	D	57)	A	B	C	D
2)	A	B	C	D	30)	A	B	C	D	58)	A	B	C	D
3)	A	B	C	D	31)	A	B	C	D	59)	A	B	C	D
4)	A	B	C	D	32)	A	B	C	D	60)	A	B	C	D
5)	A	B	C	D	33)	A	B	C	D	61)	A	B	C	D
6)	A	B	C	D	34)	A	B	C	D	62)	A	B	C	D
7)	A	B	C	D	35)	A	B	C	D	63)	A	B	C	D
8)	A	B	C	D	36)	A	B	C	D	64)	A	B	C	D
9)	A	B	C	D	37)	A	B	C	D	65)	A	B	C	D
10)	A	B	C	D	38)	A	B	C	D	66)	A	B	C	D
11)	A	B	C	D	39)	A	B	C	D	67)	A	B	C	D
12)	A	B	C	D	40)	A	B	C	D	68)	A	B	C	D
13)	A	B	C	D	41)	A	B	C	D	69)	A	B	C	D
14)	A	B	C	D	42)	A	B	C	D	70)	A	B	C	D
15)	A	B	C	D	43)	A	B	C	D	71)	A	B	C	D
16)	A	B	C	D	44)	A	B	C	D	72)	A	B	C	D
17)	A	B	C	D	45)	A	B	C	D	73)	A	B	C	D
18)	A	B	C	D	46)	A	B	C	D	74)	A	B	C	D
19)	A	B	C	D	47)	A	B	C	D	75)	A	B	C	D
20)	A	B	C	D	48)	A	B	C	D	76)	A	B	C	D
21)	A	B	C	D	49)	A	B	C	D	77)	A	B	C	D
22)	A	B	C	D	50)	A	B	C	D	78)	A	B	C	D
23)	A	B	C	D	51)	A	B	C	D	79)	A	B	C	D
24)	A	B	C	D	52)	A	B	C	D	80)	A	B	C	D
25)	A	B	C	D	53)	A	B	C	D	81)	A	B	C	D
26)	A	B	C	D	54)	A	B	C	D	82)	A	B	C	D
27)	A	B	C	D	55)	A	B	C	D	83)	A	B	C	D
28)	A	B	C	D	56)	A	B	C	D	84)	A	B	C	D

85)	A	B	C	D	116)	A	B	C	D	147)	A	B	C	D
86)	A	B	C	D	117)	A	B	C	D	148)	A	B	C	D
87)	A	B	C	D	118)	A	B	C	D	149)	A	B	C	D
88)	A	B	C	D	119)	A	B	C	D	150)	A	B	C	D
89)	A	B	C	D	120)	A	B	C	D					
90)	A	B	C	D	121)	A	B	C	D					
91)	A	B	C	D	122)	A	B	C	D					
92)	A	B	C	D	123)	A	B	C	D					
93)	A	B	C	D	124)	A	B	C	D					
94)	A	B	C	D	125)	A	B	C	D					
95)	A	B	C	D	126)	A	B	C	D					
96)	A	B	C	D	127)	A	B	C	D					
97)	A	B	C	D	128)	A	B	C	D					
98)	A	B	C	D	129)	A	B	C	D					
99)	A	B	C	D	130)	A	B	C	D					
100)	A	B	C	D	131)	A	B	C	D					
101)	A	B	C	D	132)	A	B	C	D					
102)	A	B	C	D	133)	A	B	C	D					
103)	A	B	C	D	134)	A	B	C	D					
104)	A	B	C	D	135)	A	B	C	D					
105)	A	B	C	D	136)	A	B	C	D					
106)	A	B	C	D	137)	A	B	C	D					
107)	A	B	C	D	138)	A	B	C	D					
108)	A	B	C	D	139)	A	B	C	D					
109)	A	B	C	D	140)	A	B	C	D					
110)	A	B	C	D	141)	A	B	C	D					
111)	A	B	C	D	142)	A	B	C	D					
112)	A	B	C	D	143)	A	B	C	D					
113)	A	B	C	D	144)	A	B	C	D					
114)	A	B	C	D	145)	A	B	C	D					
115)	A	B	C	D	146)	A	B	C	D					

Scoring Sheet 2   (tear our for easy use)

1) A B C D	31) A B C D	61) A B C D
2) A B C D	32) A B C D	62) A B C D
3) A B C D	33) A B C D	63) A B C D
4) A B C D	34) A B C D	64) A B C D
5) A B C D	35) A B C D	65) A B C D
6) A B C D	36) A B C D	66) A B C D
7) A B C D	37) A B C D	67) A B C D
8) A B C D	38) A B C D	68) A B C D
9) A B C D	39) A B C D	69) A B C D
10) A B C D	40) A B C D	70) A B C D
11) A B C D	41) A B C D	71) A B C D
12) A B C D	42) A B C D	72) A B C D
13) A B C D	43) A B C D	73) A B C D
14) A B C D	44) A B C D	74) A B C D
15) A B C D	45) A B C D	75) A B C D
16) A B C D	46) A B C D	76) A B C D
17) A B C D	47) A B C D	77) A B C D
18) A B C D	48) A B C D	78) A B C D
19) A B C D	49) A B C D	79) A B C D
20) A B C D	50) A B C D	80) A B C D
21) A B C D	51) A B C D	81) A B C D
22) A B C D	52) A B C D	82) A B C D
23) A B C D	53) A B C D	83) A B C D
24) A B C D	54) A B C D	84) A B C D
25) A B C D	55) A B C D	85) A B C D
26) A B C D	56) A B C D	86) A B C D
27) A B C D	57) A B C D	87) A B C D
28) A B C D	58) A B C D	88) A B C D
29) A B C D	59) A B C D	89) A B C D
30) A B C D	60) A B C D	90) A B C D

91) A B C D
92) A B C D
93) A B C D
94) A B C D
95) A B C D
96) A B C D
97) A B C D
98) A B C D
99) A B C D
100) A B C D
101) A B C D
102) A B C D
103) A B C D
104) A B C D
105) A B C D
106) A B C D
107) A B C D
108) A B C D
109) A B C D
110) A B C D
111) A B C D
112) A B C D
113) A B C D
114) A B C D
115) A B C D
116) A B C D
117) A B C D
118) A B C D
119) A B C D
120) A B C D
121) A B C D

122) A B C D
123) A B C D
124) A B C D
125) A B C D
126) A B C D
127) A B C D
128) A B C D
129) A B C D
130) A B C D
131) A B C D
132) A B C D
133) A B C D
134) A B C D
135) A B C D
136) A B C D
137) A B C D
138) A B C D
139) A B C D
140) A B C D
141) A B C D
142) A B C D
143) A B C D
144) A B C D
145) A B C D
146) A B C D
147) A B C D
148) A B C D
149) A B C D
150) A B C D

Scoring Sheet 3

(tear our for easy use)

1)	A B C D	30) A B C D	59) A B C D
2)	A B C D	31) A B C D	60) A B C D
3)	A B C D	32) A B C D	61) A B C D
4)	A B C D	33) A B C D	62) A B C D
5)	A B C D	34) A B C D	63) A B C D
6)	A B C D	35) A B C D	64) A B C D
7)	A B C D	36) A B C D	65) A B C D
8)	A B C D	37) A B C D	66) A B C D
9)	A B C D	38) A B C D	67) A B C D
10)	A B C D	39) A B C D	68) A B C D
11)	A B C D	40) A B C D	69) A B C D
12)	A B C D	41) A B C D	70) A B C D
13)	A B C D	42) A B C D	71) A B C D
14)	A B C D	43) A B C D	72) A B C D
15)	A B C D	44) A B C D	73) A B C D
16)	A B C D	45) A B C D	74) A B C D
17)	A B C D	46) A B C D	75) A B C D
18)	A B C D	47) A B C D	76) A B C D
19)	A B C D	48) A B C D	77) A B C D
20)	A B C D	49) A B C D	78) A B C D
21)	A B C D	50) A B C D	79) A B C D
22)	A B C D	51) A B C D	80) A B C D
23)	A B C D	52) A B C D	81) A B C D
24)	A B C D	53) A B C D	82) A B C D
25)	A B C D	54) A B C D	83) A B C D
26)	A B C D	55) A B C D	84) A B C D
27)	A B C D	56) A B C D	85) A B C D
28)	A B C D	57) A B C D	86) A B C D
29)	A B C D	58) A B C D	87) A B C D

88)	A	B	C	D		119)	A	B	C	D		150)	A	B	C	D
89)	A	B	C	D		120)	A	B	C	D						
90)	A	B	C	D		121)	A	B	C	D						
91)	A	B	C	D		122)	A	B	C	D						
92)	A	B	C	D		123)	A	B	C	D						
93)	A	B	C	D		124)	A	B	C	D						
94)	A	B	C	D		125)	A	B	C	D						
95)	A	B	C	D		126)	A	B	C	D						
96)	A	B	C	D		127)	A	B	C	D						
97)	A	B	C	D		128)	A	B	C	D						
98)	A	B	C	D		129)	A	B	C	D						
99)	A	B	C	D		130)	A	B	C	D						
100)	A	B	C	D		131)	A	B	C	D						
101)	A	B	C	D		132)	A	B	C	D						
102)	A	B	C	D		133)	A	B	C	D						
103)	A	B	C	D		134)	A	B	C	D						
104)	A	B	C	D		135)	A	B	C	D						
105)	A	B	C	D		136)	A	B	C	D						
106)	A	B	C	D		137)	A	B	C	D						
107)	A	B	C	D		138)	A	B	C	D						
108)	A	B	C	D		139)	A	B	C	D						
109)	A	B	C	D		140)	A	B	C	D						
110)	A	B	C	D		141)	A	B	C	D						
111)	A	B	C	D		142)	A	B	C	D						
112)	A	B	C	D		143)	A	B	C	D						
113)	A	B	C	D		144)	A	B	C	D						
114)	A	B	C	D		145)	A	B	C	D						
115)	A	B	C	D		146)	A	B	C	D						
116)	A	B	C	D		147)	A	B	C	D						
117)	A	B	C	D		148)	A	B	C	D						
118)	A	B	C	D		149)	A	B	C	D						

Scoring Sheet 4 (tear our for easy use)

1)	A B C D	30)	A B C D	59)	A B C D
2)	A B C D	31)	A B C D	60)	A B C D
3)	A B C D	32)	A B C D	61)	A B C D
4)	A B C D	33)	A B C D	62)	A B C D
5)	A B C D	34)	A B C D	63)	A B C D
6)	A B C D	35)	A B C D	64)	A B C D
7)	A B C D	36)	A B C D	65)	A B C D
8)	A B C D	37)	A B C D	66)	A B C D
9)	A B C D	38)	A B C D	67)	A B C D
10)	A B C D	39)	A B C D	68)	A B C D
11)	A B C D	40)	A B C D	69)	A B C D
12)	A B C D	41)	A B C D	70)	A B C D
13)	A B C D	42)	A B C D	71)	A B C D
14)	A B C D	43)	A B C D	72)	A B C D
15)	A B C D	44)	A B C D	73)	A B C D
16)	A B C D	45)	A B C D	74)	A B C D
17)	A B C D	46)	A B C D	75)	A B C D
18)	A B C D	47)	A B C D	76)	A B C D
19)	A B C D	48)	A B C D	77)	A B C D
20)	A B C D	49)	A B C D	78)	A B C D
21)	A B C D	50)	A B C D	79)	A B C D
22)	A B C D	51)	A B C D	80)	A B C D
23)	A B C D	52)	A B C D	81)	A B C D
24)	A B C D	53)	A B C D	82)	A B C D
25)	A B C D	54)	A B C D	83)	A B C D
26)	A B C D	55)	A B C D	84)	A B C D
27)	A B C D	56)	A B C D	85)	A B C D
28)	A B C D	57)	A B C D	86)	A B C D
29)	A B C D	58)	A B C D	87)	A B C D

88)	A	B	C	D	119)	A	B	C	D	150)	A	B	C	D
89)	A	B	C	D	120)	A	B	C	D
90)	A	B	C	D	121)	A	B	C	D
91)	A	B	C	D	122)	A	B	C	D
92)	A	B	C	D	123)	A	B	C	D
93)	A	B	C	D	124)	A	B	C	D
94)	A	B	C	D	125)	A	B	C	D
95)	A	B	C	D	126)	A	B	C	D
96)	A	B	C	D	127)	A	B	C	D
97)	A	B	C	D	128)	A	B	C	D
98)	A	B	C	D	129)	A	B	C	D
99)	A	B	C	D	130)	A	B	C	D
100)	A	B	C	D	131)	A	B	C	D
101)	A	B	C	D	132)	A	B	C	D
102)	A	B	C	D	133)	A	B	C	D
103)	A	B	C	D	134)	A	B	C	D
104)	A	B	C	D	135)	A	B	C	D
105)	A	B	C	D	136)	A	B	C	D
106)	A	B	C	D	137)	A	B	C	D
107)	A	B	C	D	138)	A	B	C	D
108)	A	B	C	D	139)	A	B	C	D
109)	A	B	C	D	140)	A	B	C	D
110)	A	B	C	D	141)	A	B	C	D
111)	A	B	C	D	142)	A	B	C	D
112)	A	B	C	D	143)	A	B	C	D
113)	A	B	C	D	144)	A	B	C	D
114)	A	B	C	D	145)	A	B	C	D
115)	A	B	C	D	146)	A	B	C	D
116)	A	B	C	D	147)	A	B	C	D
117)	A	B	C	D	148)	A	B	C	D
118)	A	B	C	D	149)	A	B	C	D

Scoring Sheet 5 (tear our for easy use)

1)	A	B	C	D	30)	A	B	C	D	59)	A	B	C	D
2)	A	B	C	D	31)	A	B	C	D	60)	A	B	C	D
3)	A	B	C	D	32)	A	B	C	D	61)	A	B	C	D
4)	A	B	C	D	33)	A	B	C	D	62)	A	B	C	D
5)	A	B	C	D	34)	A	B	C	D	63)	A	B	C	D
6)	A	B	C	D	35)	A	B	C	D	64)	A	B	C	D
7)	A	B	C	D	36)	A	B	C	D	65)	A	B	C	D
8)	A	B	C	D	37)	A	B	C	D	66)	A	B	C	D
9)	A	B	C	D	38)	A	B	C	D	67)	A	B	C	D
10)	A	B	C	D	39)	A	B	C	D	68)	A	B	C	D
11)	A	B	C	D	40)	A	B	C	D	69)	A	B	C	D
12)	A	B	C	D	41)	A	B	C	D	70)	A	B	C	D
13)	A	B	C	D	42)	A	B	C	D	71)	A	B	C	D
14)	A	B	C	D	43)	A	B	C	D	72)	A	B	C	D
15)	A	B	C	D	44)	A	B	C	D	73)	A	B	C	D
16)	A	B	C	D	45)	A	B	C	D	74)	A	B	C	D
17)	A	B	C	D	46)	A	B	C	D	75)	A	B	C	D
18)	A	B	C	D	47)	A	B	C	D	76)	A	B	C	D
19)	A	B	C	D	48)	A	B	C	D	77)	A	B	C	D
20)	A	B	C	D	49)	A	B	C	D	78)	A	B	C	D
21)	A	B	C	D	50)	A	B	C	D	79)	A	B	C	D
22)	A	B	C	D	51)	A	B	C	D	80)	A	B	C	D
23)	A	B	C	D	52)	A	B	C	D	81)	A	B	C	D
24)	A	B	C	D	53)	A	B	C	D	82)	A	B	C	D
25)	A	B	C	D	54)	A	B	C	D	83)	A	B	C	D
26)	A	B	C	D	55)	A	B	C	D	84)	A	B	C	D
27)	A	B	C	D	56)	A	B	C	D	85)	A	B	C	D
28)	A	B	C	D	57)	A	B	C	D	86)	A	B	C	D
29)	A	B	C	D	58)	A	B	C	D	87)	A	B	C	D

88)	A	B	C	D	119)	A	B	C	D	150)	A	B	C	D
89)	A	B	C	D	120)	A	B	C	D					
90)	A	B	C	D	121)	A	B	C	D					
91)	A	B	C	D	122)	A	B	C	D					
92)	A	B	C	D	123)	A	B	C	D					
93)	A	B	C	D	124)	A	B	C	D					
94)	A	B	C	D	125)	A	B	C	D					
95)	A	B	C	D	126)	A	B	C	D					
96)	A	B	C	D	127)	A	B	C	D					
97)	A	B	C	D	128)	A	B	C	D					
98)	A	B	C	D	129)	A	B	C	D					
99)	A	B	C	D	130)	A	B	C	D					
100)	A	B	C	D	131)	A	B	C	D					
101)	A	B	C	D	132)	A	B	C	D					
102)	A	B	C	D	133)	A	B	C	D					
103)	A	B	C	D	134)	A	B	C	D					
104)	A	B	C	D	135)	A	B	C	D					
105)	A	B	C	D	136)	A	B	C	D					
106)	A	B	C	D	137)	A	B	C	D					
107)	A	B	C	D	138)	A	B	C	D					
108)	A	B	C	D	139)	A	B	C	D					
109)	A	B	C	D	140)	A	B	C	D					
110)	A	B	C	D	141)	A	B	C	D					
111)	A	B	C	D	142)	A	B	C	D					
112)	A	B	C	D	143)	A	B	C	D					
113)	A	B	C	D	144)	A	B	C	D					
114)	A	B	C	D	145)	A	B	C	D					
115)	A	B	C	D	146)	A	B	C	D					
116)	A	B	C	D	147)	A	B	C	D					
117)	A	B	C	D	148)	A	B	C	D					
118)	A	B	C	D	149)	A	B	C	D					

Scoring Sheet 6   (tear our for easy use)

1)	A B C D	30)	A B C D	59)	A B C D
2)	A B C D	31)	A B C D	60)	A B C D
3)	A B C D	32)	A B C D	61)	A B C D
4)	A B C D	33)	A B C D	62)	A B C D
5)	A B C D	34)	A B C D	63)	A B C D
6)	A B C D	35)	A B C D	64)	A B C D
7)	A B C D	36)	A B C D	65)	A B C D
8)	A B C D	37)	A B C D	66)	A B C D
9)	A B C D	38)	A B C D	67)	A B C D
10)	A B C D	39)	A B C D	68)	A B C D
11)	A B C D	40)	A B C D	69)	A B C D
12)	A B C D	41)	A B C D	70)	A B C D
13)	A B C D	42)	A B C D	71)	A B C D
14)	A B C D	43)	A B C D	72)	A B C D
15)	A B C D	44)	A B C D	73)	A B C D
16)	A B C D	45)	A B C D	74)	A B C D
17)	A B C D	46)	A B C D	75)	A B C D
18)	A B C D	47)	A B C D	76)	A B C D
19)	A B C D	48)	A B C D	77)	A B C D
20)	A B C D	49)	A B C D	78)	A B C D
21)	A B C D	50)	A B C D	79)	A B C D
22)	A B C D	51)	A B C D	80)	A B C D
23)	A B C D	52)	A B C D	81)	A B C D
24)	A B C D	53)	A B C D	82)	A B C D
25)	A B C D	54)	A B C D	83)	A B C D
26)	A B C D	55)	A B C D	84)	A B C D
27)	A B C D	56)	A B C D	85)	A B C D
28)	A B C D	57)	A B C D	86)	A B C D
29)	A B C D	58)	A B C D	87)	A B C D

88)	A	B	C	D	119)	A	B	C	D	150)	A	B	C	D
89)	A	B	C	D	120)	A	B	C	D
90)	A	B	C	D	121)	A	B	C	D
91)	A	B	C	D	122)	A	B	C	D
92)	A	B	C	D	123)	A	B	C	D
93)	A	B	C	D	124)	A	B	C	D
94)	A	B	C	D	125)	A	B	C	D
95)	A	B	C	D	126)	A	B	C	D
96)	A	B	C	D	127)	A	B	C	D
97)	A	B	C	D	128)	A	B	C	D
98)	A	B	C	D	129)	A	B	C	D
99)	A	B	C	D	130)	A	B	C	D
100)	A	B	C	D	131)	A	B	C	D
101)	A	B	C	D	132)	A	B	C	D
102)	A	B	C	D	133)	A	B	C	D
103)	A	B	C	D	134)	A	B	C	D
104)	A	B	C	D	135)	A	B	C	D
105)	A	B	C	D	136)	A	B	C	D
106)	A	B	C	D	137)	A	B	C	D
107)	A	B	C	D	138)	A	B	C	D
108)	A	B	C	D	139)	A	B	C	D
109)	A	B	C	D	140)	A	B	C	D
110)	A	B	C	D	141)	A	B	C	D
111)	A	B	C	D	142)	A	B	C	D
112)	A	B	C	D	143)	A	B	C	D
113)	A	B	C	D	144)	A	B	C	D
114)	A	B	C	D	145)	A	B	C	D
115)	A	B	C	D	146)	A	B	C	D
116)	A	B	C	D	147)	A	B	C	D
117)	A	B	C	D	148)	A	B	C	D
118)	A	B	C	D	149)	A	B	C	D

Scoring Sheet 7   (tear our for easy use)

1) A B C D	30) A B C D	59) A B C D
2) A B C D	31) A B C D	60) A B C D
3) A B C D	32) A B C D	61) A B C D
4) A B C D	33) A B C D	62) A B C D
5) A B C D	34) A B C D	63) A B C D
6) A B C D	35) A B C D	64) A B C D
7) A B C D	36) A B C D	65) A B C D
8) A B C D	37) A B C D	66) A B C D
9) A B C D	38) A B C D	67) A B C D
10) A B C D	39) A B C D	68) A B C D
11) A B C D	40) A B C D	69) A B C D
12) A B C D	41) A B C D	70) A B C D
13) A B C D	42) A B C D	71) A B C D
14) A B C D	43) A B C D	72) A B C D
15) A B C D	44) A B C D	73) A B C D
16) A B C D	45) A B C D	74) A B C D
17) A B C D	46) A B C D	75) A B C D
18) A B C D	47) A B C D	76) A B C D
19) A B C D	48) A B C D	77) A B C D
20) A B C D	49) A B C D	78) A B C D
21) A B C D	50) A B C D	79) A B C D
22) A B C D	51) A B C D	80) A B C D
23) A B C D	52) A B C D	81) A B C D
24) A B C D	53) A B C D	82) A B C D
25) A B C D	54) A B C D	83) A B C D
26) A B C D	55) A B C D	84) A B C D
27) A B C D	56) A B C D	85) A B C D
28) A B C D	57) A B C D	86) A B C D
29) A B C D	58) A B C D	87) A B C D

88)	A	B	C	D	119)	A	B	C	D	150)	A	B	C	D
89)	A	B	C	D	120)	A	B	C	D					
90)	A	B	C	D	121)	A	B	C	D					
91)	A	B	C	D	122)	A	B	C	D					
92)	A	B	C	D	123)	A	B	C	D					
93)	A	B	C	D	124)	A	B	C	D					
94)	A	B	C	D	125)	A	B	C	D					
95)	A	B	C	D	126)	A	B	C	D					
96)	A	B	C	D	127)	A	B	C	D					
97)	A	B	C	D	128)	A	B	C	D					
98)	A	B	C	D	129)	A	B	C	D					
99)	A	B	C	D	130)	A	B	C	D					
100)	A	B	C	D	131)	A	B	C	D					
101)	A	B	C	D	132)	A	B	C	D					
102)	A	B	C	D	133)	A	B	C	D					
103)	A	B	C	D	134)	A	B	C	D					
104)	A	B	C	D	135)	A	B	C	D					
105)	A	B	C	D	136)	A	B	C	D					
106)	A	B	C	D	137)	A	B	C	D					
107)	A	B	C	D	138)	A	B	C	D					
108)	A	B	C	D	139)	A	B	C	D					
109)	A	B	C	D	140)	A	B	C	D					
110)	A	B	C	D	141)	A	B	C	D					
111)	A	B	C	D	142)	A	B	C	D					
112)	A	B	C	D	143)	A	B	C	D					
113)	A	B	C	D	144)	A	B	C	D					
114)	A	B	C	D	145)	A	B	C	D					
115)	A	B	C	D	146)	A	B	C	D					
116)	A	B	C	D	147)	A	B	C	D					
117)	A	B	C	D	148)	A	B	C	D					
118)	A	B	C	D	149)	A	B	C	D					

Scoring Sheet 8 (tear our for easy use)

1)	A B C D	30) A B C D	59) A B C D
2)	A B C D	31) A B C D	60) A B C D
3)	A B C D	32) A B C D	61) A B C D
4)	A B C D	33) A B C D	62) A B C D
5)	A B C D	34) A B C D	63) A B C D
6)	A B C D	35) A B C D	64) A B C D
7)	A B C D	36) A B C D	65) A B C D
8)	A B C D	37) A B C D	66) A B C D
9)	A B C D	38) A B C D	67) A B C D
10)	A B C D	39) A B C D	68) A B C D
11)	A B C D	40) A B C D	69) A B C D
12)	A B C D	41) A B C D	70) A B C D
13)	A B C D	42) A B C D	71) A B C D
14)	A B C D	43) A B C D	72) A B C D
15)	A B C D	44) A B C D	73) A B C D
16)	A B C D	45) A B C D	74) A B C D
17)	A B C D	46) A B C D	75) A B C D
18)	A B C D	47) A B C D	76) A B C D
19)	A B C D	48) A B C D	77) A B C D
20)	A B C D	49) A B C D	78) A B C D
21)	A B C D	50) A B C D	79) A B C D
22)	A B C D	51) A B C D	80) A B C D
23)	A B C D	52) A B C D	81) A B C D
24)	A B C D	53) A B C D	82) A B C D
25)	A B C D	54) A B C D	83) A B C D
26)	A B C D	55) A B C D	84) A B C D
27)	A B C D	56) A B C D	85) A B C D
28)	A B C D	57) A B C D	86) A B C D
29)	A B C D	58) A B C D	87) A B C D

88)	A	B	C	D	119)	A	B	C	D	150)	A	B	C	D
89)	A	B	C	D	120)	A	B	C	D					
90)	A	B	C	D	121)	A	B	C	D					
91)	A	B	C	D	122)	A	B	C	D					
92)	A	B	C	D	123)	A	B	C	D					
93)	A	B	C	D	124)	A	B	C	D					
94)	A	B	C	D	125)	A	B	C	D					
95)	A	B	C	D	126)	A	B	C	D					
96)	A	B	C	D	127)	A	B	C	D					
97)	A	B	C	D	128)	A	B	C	D					
98)	A	B	C	D	129)	A	B	C	D					
99)	A	B	C	D	130)	A	B	C	D					
100)	A	B	C	D	131)	A	B	C	D					
101)	A	B	C	D	132)	A	B	C	D					
102)	A	B	C	D	133)	A	B	C	D					
103)	A	B	C	D	134)	A	B	C	D					
104)	A	B	C	D	135)	A	B	C	D					
105)	A	B	C	D	136)	A	B	C	D					
106)	A	B	C	D	137)	A	B	C	D					
107)	A	B	C	D	138)	A	B	C	D					
108)	A	B	C	D	139)	A	B	C	D					
109)	A	B	C	D	140)	A	B	C	D					
110)	A	B	C	D	141)	A	B	C	D					
111)	A	B	C	D	142)	A	B	C	D					
112)	A	B	C	D	143)	A	B	C	D					
113)	A	B	C	D	144)	A	B	C	D					
114)	A	B	C	D	145)	A	B	C	D					
115)	A	B	C	D	146)	A	B	C	D					
116)	A	B	C	D	147)	A	B	C	D					
117)	A	B	C	D	148)	A	B	C	D					
118)	A	B	C	D	149)	A	B	C	D					

Scoring Sheet 9   (tear our for easy use)

1)	A	B	C	D
2)	A	B	C	D
3)	A	B	C	D
4)	A	B	C	D
5)	A	B	C	D

1)   A   B   C   D   30)   A   B   C   D   59)   A   B   C   D
2)   A   B   C   D   31)   A   B   C   D   60)   A   B   C   D
3)   A   B   C   D   32)   A   B   C   D   61)   A   B   C   D
4)   A   B   C   D   33)   A   B   C   D   62)   A   B   C   D
5)   A   B   C   D   34)   A   B   C   D   63)   A   B   C   D
6)   A   B   C   D   35)   A   B   C   D   64)   A   B   C   D
7)   A   B   C   D   36)   A   B   C   D   65)   A   B   C   D
8)   A   B   C   D   37)   A   B   C   D   66)   A   B   C   D
9)   A   B   C   D   38)   A   B   C   D   67)   A   B   C   D
10) A   B   C   D   39)   A   B   C   D   68)   A   B   C   D
11) A   B   C   D   40)   A   B   C   D   69)   A   B   C   D
12) A   B   C   D   41)   A   B   C   D   70)   A   B   C   D
13) A   B   C   D   42)   A   B   C   D   71)   A   B   C   D
14) A   B   C   D   43)   A   B   C   D   72)   A   B   C   D
15) A   B   C   D   44)   A   B   C   D   73)   A   B   C   D
16) A   B   C   D   45)   A   B   C   D   74)   A   B   C   D
17) A   B   C   D   46)   A   B   C   D   75)   A   B   C   D
18) A   B   C   D   47)   A   B   C   D   76)   A   B   C   D
19) A   B   C   D   48)   A   B   C   D   77)   A   B   C   D
20) A   B   C   D   49)   A   B   C   D   78)   A   B   C   D
21) A   B   C   D   50)   A   B   C   D   79)   A   B   C   D
22) A   B   C   D   51)   A   B   C   D   80)   A   B   C   D
23) A   B   C   D   52)   A   B   C   D   81)   A   B   C   D
24) A   B   C   D   53)   A   B   C   D   82)   A   B   C   D
25) A   B   C   D   54)   A   B   C   D   83)   A   B   C   D
26) A   B   C   D   55)   A   B   C   D   84)   A   B   C   D
27) A   B   C   D   56)   A   B   C   D   85)   A   B   C   D
28) A   B   C   D   57)   A   B   C   D   86)   A   B   C   D
29) A   B   C   D   58)   A   B   C   D   87)   A   B   C   D

88)	A	B	C	D	119)	A	B	C	D	150)	A	B	C	D
89)	A	B	C	D	120)	A	B	C	D					
90)	A	B	C	D	121)	A	B	C	D					
91)	A	B	C	D	122)	A	B	C	D					
92)	A	B	C	D	123)	A	B	C	D					
93)	A	B	C	D	124)	A	B	C	D					
94)	A	B	C	D	125)	A	B	C	D					
95)	A	B	C	D	126)	A	B	C	D					
96)	A	B	C	D	127)	A	B	C	D					
97)	A	B	C	D	128)	A	B	C	D					
98)	A	B	C	D	129)	A	B	C	D					
99)	A	B	C	D	130)	A	B	C	D					
100)	A	B	C	D	131)	A	B	C	D					
101)	A	B	C	D	132)	A	B	C	D					
102)	A	B	C	D	133)	A	B	C	D					
103)	A	B	C	D	134)	A	B	C	D					
104)	A	B	C	D	135)	A	B	C	D					
105)	A	B	C	D	136)	A	B	C	D					
106)	A	B	C	D	137)	A	B	C	D					
107)	A	B	C	D	138)	A	B	C	D					
108)	A	B	C	D	139)	A	B	C	D					
109)	A	B	C	D	140)	A	B	C	D					
110)	A	B	C	D	141)	A	B	C	D					
111)	A	B	C	D	142)	A	B	C	D					
112)	A	B	C	D	143)	A	B	C	D					
113)	A	B	C	D	144)	A	B	C	D					
114)	A	B	C	D	145)	A	B	C	D					
115)	A	B	C	D	146)	A	B	C	D					
116)	A	B	C	D	147)	A	B	C	D					
117)	A	B	C	D	148)	A	B	C	D					
118)	A	B	C	D	149)	A	B	C	D					

Scoring Sheet 10   (tear our for easy use)

1) A B C D	30) A B C D	59) A B C D
2) A B C D	31) A B C D	60) A B C D
3) A B C D	32) A B C D	61) A B C D
4) A B C D	33) A B C D	62) A B C D
5) A B C D	34) A B C D	63) A B C D
6) A B C D	35) A B C D	64) A B C D
7) A B C D	36) A B C D	65) A B C D
8) A B C D	37) A B C D	66) A B C D
9) A B C D	38) A B C D	67) A B C D
10) A B C D	39) A B C D	68) A B C D
11) A B C D	40) A B C D	69) A B C D
12) A B C D	41) A B C D	70) A B C D
13) A B C D	42) A B C D	71) A B C D
14) A B C D	43) A B C D	72) A B C D
15) A B C D	44) A B C D	73) A B C D
16) A B C D	45) A B C D	74) A B C D
17) A B C D	46) A B C D	75) A B C D
18) A B C D	47) A B C D	76) A B C D
19) A B C D	48) A B C D	77) A B C D
20) A B C D	49) A B C D	78) A B C D
21) A B C D	50) A B C D	79) A B C D
22) A B C D	51) A B C D	80) A B C D
23) A B C D	52) A B C D	81) A B C D
24) A B C D	53) A B C D	82) A B C D
25) A B C D	54) A B C D	83) A B C D
26) A B C D	55) A B C D	84) A B C D
27) A B C D	56) A B C D	85) A B C D
28) A B C D	57) A B C D	86) A B C D
29) A B C D	58) A B C D	87) A B C D

88)	A	B	C	D		119)	A	B	C	D		150)	A	B	C	D
89)	A	B	C	D		120)	A	B	C	D						
90)	A	B	C	D		121)	A	B	C	D						
91)	A	B	C	D		122)	A	B	C	D						
92)	A	B	C	D		123)	A	B	C	D						
93)	A	B	C	D		124)	A	B	C	D						
94)	A	B	C	D		125)	A	B	C	D						
95)	A	B	C	D		126)	A	B	C	D						
96)	A	B	C	D		127)	A	B	C	D						
97)	A	B	C	D		128)	A	B	C	D						
98)	A	B	C	D		129)	A	B	C	D						
99)	A	B	C	D		130)	A	B	C	D						
100)	A	B	C	D		131)	A	B	C	D						
101)	A	B	C	D		132)	A	B	C	D						
102)	A	B	C	D		133)	A	B	C	D						
103)	A	B	C	D		134)	A	B	C	D						
104)	A	B	C	D		135)	A	B	C	D						
105)	A	B	C	D		136)	A	B	C	D						
106)	A	B	C	D		137)	A	B	C	D						
107)	A	B	C	D		138)	A	B	C	D						
108)	A	B	C	D		139)	A	B	C	D						
109)	A	B	C	D		140)	A	B	C	D						
110)	A	B	C	D		141)	A	B	C	D						
111)	A	B	C	D		142)	A	B	C	D						
112)	A	B	C	D		143)	A	B	C	D						
113)	A	B	C	D		144)	A	B	C	D						
114)	A	B	C	D		145)	A	B	C	D						
115)	A	B	C	D		146)	A	B	C	D						
116)	A	B	C	D		147)	A	B	C	D						
117)	A	B	C	D		148)	A	B	C	D						
118)	A	B	C	D		149)	A	B	C	D						

Scoring Sheet 11   (tear our for easy use)

1) A B C D		30) A B C D		59) A B C D
2) A B C D		31) A B C D		60) A B C D
3) A B C D		32) A B C D		61) A B C D
4) A B C D		33) A B C D		62) A B C D
5) A B C D		34) A B C D		63) A B C D
6) A B C D		35) A B C D		64) A B C D
7) A B C D		36) A B C D		65) A B C D
8) A B C D		37) A B C D		66) A B C D
9) A B C D		38) A B C D		67) A B C D
10) A B C D		39) A B C D		68) A B C D
11) A B C D		40) A B C D		69) A B C D
12) A B C D		41) A B C D		70) A B C D
13) A B C D		42) A B C D		71) A B C D
14) A B C D		43) A B C D		72) A B C D
15) A B C D		44) A B C D		73) A B C D
16) A B C D		45) A B C D		74) A B C D
17) A B C D		46) A B C D		75) A B C D
18) A B C D		47) A B C D		76) A B C D
19) A B C D		48) A B C D		77) A B C D
20) A B C D		49) A B C D		78) A B C D
21) A B C D		50) A B C D		79) A B C D
22) A B C D		51) A B C D		80) A B C D
23) A B C D		52) A B C D		81) A B C D
24) A B C D		53) A B C D		82) A B C D
25) A B C D		54) A B C D		83) A B C D
26) A B C D		55) A B C D		84) A B C D
27) A B C D		56) A B C D		85) A B C D
28) A B C D		57) A B C D		86) A B C D
29) A B C D		58) A B C D		87) A B C D

88) A B C D	119) A B C D	150) A B C D
89) A B C D	120) A B C D	
90) A B C D	121) A B C D	
91) A B C D	122) A B C D	
92) A B C D	123) A B C D	
93) A B C D	124) A B C D	
94) A B C D	125) A B C D	
95) A B C D	126) A B C D	
96) A B C D	127) A B C D	
97) A B C D	128) A B C D	
98) A B C D	129) A B C D	
99) A B C D	130) A B C D	
100) A B C D	131) A B C D	
101) A B C D	132) A B C D	
102) A B C D	133) A B C D	
103) A B C D	134) A B C D	
104) A B C D	135) A B C D	
105) A B C D	136) A B C D	
106) A B C D	137) A B C D	
107) A B C D	138) A B C D	
108) A B C D	139) A B C D	
109) A B C D	140) A B C D	
110) A B C D	141) A B C D	
111) A B C D	142) A B C D	
112) A B C D	143) A B C D	
113) A B C D	144) A B C D	
114) A B C D	145) A B C D	
115) A B C D	146) A B C D	
116) A B C D	147) A B C D	
117) A B C D	148) A B C D	
118) A B C D	149) A B C D	

Scoring Sheet 12   (tear our for easy use)

1)	A	B	C	D	30)	A	B	C	D	59)	A	B	C	D
2)	A	B	C	D	31)	A	B	C	D	60)	A	B	C	D
3)	A	B	C	D	32)	A	B	C	D	61)	A	B	C	D
4)	A	B	C	D	33)	A	B	C	D	62)	A	B	C	D
5)	A	B	C	D	34)	A	B	C	D	63)	A	B	C	D
6)	A	B	C	D	35)	A	B	C	D	64)	A	B	C	D
7)	A	B	C	D	36)	A	B	C	D	65)	A	B	C	D
8)	A	B	C	D	37)	A	B	C	D	66)	A	B	C	D
9)	A	B	C	D	38)	A	B	C	D	67)	A	B	C	D
10)	A	B	C	D	39)	A	B	C	D	68)	A	B	C	D
11)	A	B	C	D	40)	A	B	C	D	69)	A	B	C	D
12)	A	B	C	D	41)	A	B	C	D	70)	A	B	C	D
13)	A	B	C	D	42)	A	B	C	D	71)	A	B	C	D
14)	A	B	C	D	43)	A	B	C	D	72)	A	B	C	D
15)	A	B	C	D	44)	A	B	C	D	73)	A	B	C	D
16)	A	B	C	D	45)	A	B	C	D	74)	A	B	C	D
17)	A	B	C	D	46)	A	B	C	D	75)	A	B	C	D
18)	A	B	C	D	47)	A	B	C	D	76)	A	B	C	D
19)	A	B	C	D	48)	A	B	C	D	77)	A	B	C	D
20)	A	B	C	D	49)	A	B	C	D	78)	A	B	C	D
21)	A	B	C	D	50)	A	B	C	D	79)	A	B	C	D
22)	A	B	C	D	51)	A	B	C	D	80)	A	B	C	D
23)	A	B	C	D	52)	A	B	C	D	81)	A	B	C	D
24)	A	B	C	D	53)	A	B	C	D	82)	A	B	C	D
25)	A	B	C	D	54)	A	B	C	D	83)	A	B	C	D
26)	A	B	C	D	55)	A	B	C	D	84)	A	B	C	D
27)	A	B	C	D	56)	A	B	C	D	85)	A	B	C	D
28)	A	B	C	D	57)	A	B	C	D	86)	A	B	C	D
29)	A	B	C	D	58)	A	B	C	D	87)	A	B	C	D

88)	A	B	C	D	119)	A	B	C	D
89)	A	B	C	D	120)	A	B	C	D
90)	A	B	C	D	121)	A	B	C	D
91)	A	B	C	D	122)	A	B	C	D
92)	A	B	C	D	123)	A	B	C	D
93)	A	B	C	D	124)	A	B	C	D
94)	A	B	C	D	125)	A	B	C	D
95)	A	B	C	D	126)	A	B	C	D
96)	A	B	C	D	127)	A	B	C	D
97)	A	B	C	D	128)	A	B	C	D
98)	A	B	C	D	129)	A	B	C	D
99)	A	B	C	D	130)	A	B	C	D
100)	A	B	C	D	131)	A	B	C	D
101)	A	B	C	D	132)	A	B	C	D
102)	A	B	C	D	133)	A	B	C	D
103)	A	B	C	D	134)	A	B	C	D
104)	A	B	C	D	135)	A	B	C	D
105)	A	B	C	D	136)	A	B	C	D
106)	A	B	C	D	137)	A	B	C	D
107)	A	B	C	D	138)	A	B	C	D
108)	A	B	C	D	139)	A	B	C	D
109)	A	B	C	D	140)	A	B	C	D
110)	A	B	C	D	141)	A	B	C	D
111)	A	B	C	D	142)	A	B	C	D
112)	A	B	C	D	143)	A	B	C	D
113)	A	B	C	D	144)	A	B	C	D
114)	A	B	C	D	145)	A	B	C	D
115)	A	B	C	D	146)	A	B	C	D
116)	A	B	C	D	147)	A	B	C	D
117)	A	B	C	D	148)	A	B	C	D
118)	A	B	C	D	149)	A	B	C	D

150) A   B   C   D

Secrets To Reducing Exam Stress

What is Stress

Stress is a normal physical response to events that make you feel threatened or upset your balance in some way, such as situations beyond your control.

The body reacts to these situations with physical, mental, and emotional responses that all merge to create what is known as stress.

When you sense danger or events beyond your control the body's defense mechanisms kick into high gear causing a built in chain reaction of events to occur. This is natural for all of us.

Remember the first time someone reprimanded you for something you had done wrong? Not necessarily a parent or relative, but someone in school or at your place of employment where you felt threatened and began feeling stressed and nervous? That was a natural reaction to a set of circumstances that caused you to feel the effects of stress.

This can be a good thing during an emergency or other event but can also be a bad thing when you are trying to concentrate or think clearly for long periods of time, such as during an exam.

What Causes Stress and Anxiety

Stress is caused by fear, plain and simple. The fear of the unknown. The fear of failing. The fear of being unprepared. The fear of loss. The fear of an uncontrollable situation.

Anything beyond our control can cause fear or a sense of danger and this causes the body to release stress hormones, thus increasing your stress and anxiety level.

There are other factors that cause stress too including family, income, job, friends, life situations and others but the main focus of this book is stress directly attributed to exam preparation and taking an exam.

Once you learn how to reduce and manage stress for an exam you can certainly expand its uses to other areas of your life as well. As a matter of fact, I highly recommend that you do. The facts are clear, the less stress you have in your life the longer you will live and the better quality of life you will have.

What Are The Side Effects Of Stress

When stress is not controlled it can cause a significant amount of problems for people taking an exam. You have likely already experienced some of the side effects of stress including:

• Memory Problems

• Lack of Concentration

• Poor Judgement

• Negative Thoughts

• Headaches

• High Blood Pressure

• Upset Stomach

Each of these side effects can affect your exam preparation efforts and performance. As a matter of fact, in some extreme cases it can cause people to "lock up" and have difficulty even taking an exam. These cases are rare but they do exist. If you suffer from this type of reaction you know all too well how difficult it is to perform under these conditions, let alone excel or perform well enough to earn a passing grade.

So how can you control or minimize the effects of stress and even make it work for you?

Learn to Relax

Setting your mind at ease and learning how to relax can reduce stress dramatically. This is much easier said than done, however, there are different techniques to help you relax and each have there own set of benefits.

There are many different ways to relax your mind and body. Some are more difficult than others. Let's begin with an easy way to reduce even the most sever cases of stress.

Slow Breathing

When you begin to feel the effects of stress your breathing accelerates and your heart rate quickens. This is caused by adrenaline being pumped into your system from the body's reaction to a circumstance or situation.

The first thing you have to do is recognize that you are experiencing stress. After you have done that, the easiest and fastest way to reduce your stress level is to slow your breathing.

If you have ever watched a sporting event you have probably seen top athletes using this method to slow their heart rate, reduce adrenaline flow, relax their muscles, and clear their minds.

This helps them think more clearly, react more rapidly, and perform at a higher level. This is exactly what you want to do.

Top athletes do this when adrenaline is not a good thing and can effect performance.

A good example of this is golf. A golfer relies heavily on muscle memory to produce accurate and consistent golf shots. When adrenaline is introduced into their system, say during the final round of a tournament, it can cause a variation in the distance they hit the ball.

This can make them inconsistent at the very time when they need to be the most consistent.

And at the same time... with the stress level now amped up it can cause a player who normally makes sound decisions to now make questionable ones. This is strikingly similar to an exam situation.

Give this method a try. Take a deep breath and exhale slowly. Repeat this several times until your muscles are totally relaxed and your heart rate slows.

Use this method before studying and prior to and during the exam itself! It will help you think more clearly and be able to recall learned information more rapidly. This technique should be the first thing you do when you start to feel anxious or stressed.

"SOMETIMES WHEN PEOPLE ARE UNDER STRESS THEY HATE TO THINK, AND IT'S THE TIME THEY MOST NEED TO THINK."

PRESIDENT BILL CLINTON

Meditation

Please don't be intimidated by the word "meditation". It is not something to fear, rather something to embrace once you know a little more about it.

Meditation can give your mind a chance to take a much needed break, to "shut down", relax and recharge.

The biggest misconception about meditation is that it is something complex. It isn't. It is simply the process of relaxing your mind and body to give it a much needed break. This is exactly what you need to relieve stress.

Time to Meditate

Meditation does not take that long to do and it can be immensely valuable for your mind, body, and spirit. Scheduling a time to meditate is the best way to make sure it happens on a regular basis.

Set aside ten minutes prior to your scheduled study time each day to meditate. This will get you into the routine of doing it. Also schedule ten to twenty minutes prior to taking an exam to meditate when possible. It will help you relax and open your mind for better memory retention during study time and better information recall during exam time.

Meditation Exercises

Follow these simple steps to enjoy a deeper sense of relaxation.

- Sit in a relaxed position.
- Close your eyes.
- Rest your hands, palms up, on your lap.
- Breathe slowly and slightly deeper than normal.

- Concentrate on your breath coming in and going out.

- Quiet your mind. If you are thinking of something try to release the thought and concentrate on breathing again.

- As you become relaxed repeat a calming word or phrase such as "I feel calm" or "I can achieve", or even "I am the best".

- After ten minutes open your eyes slowly.

This should thoroughly relax you and give you positive thoughts and energy. Now your mind is free to accept new information when studying and ready to recall learned information more rapidly and accurately when taking an exam.

Meditation is nothing more than focused relaxation for the mind and body. Look at it this way. You rest your body six to eight hours per night. Sometimes your mind is resting but not always. So your mind doesn't get as much rest as your body does, just as everything else, it needs rest to be able to perform at a high level.

This is good for daily use, but *ultra* effective prior to exam preparation and before an actual exam.

Set Up A Routine

One of the most important actions you can take to reduce stress and anxiety is set up a study routine.

By setting up a regular study routine you remove the stress of trying to find time everyday to study. Schedule the time in advance. Commit to it and stick to it.

You know what time you have to go to work everyday... right? Why not know what time you are going to study everyday? All good habits are scheduled and repeated. Study time should be no different.

Scheduling

The best time to lay out a schedule is about a month to forty five days prior to an exam when possible. All exams are different but mapping out a consistent plan is essential. This is your way to say "this is important to me".

This will give you enough time to review all the material in a timely manner without cramming it all in at the last minute. This alone will reduce your stress level significantly as well as boost your confidence.

How Often Should You Study

A good study routine should consist of regularly scheduled short periods of uninterrupted and focused study time every day. This will give you time to absorb the information when you are alert and can concentrate fully.

Your study time should <u>not</u> consist of hours upon hours of study time in one day and then no study time for several days. This will wear you down and reduce your ability to retain and recall information.

The last minute "all nighter" is the worst thing you can do! This time should only be for a last minute review of the most difficult material.

Plodding through hundreds of pages of information the night before an exam will only deprive you of sleep you desperately need and dilute any information you have already committed to memory.

You might occasionally "luck out" on an exam this way but keep in mind how much better you could have done had you prepared the right way.

How Long Should You Study

The ideal daily study time is an hour to two hours per day maximum! This will ultimately depend on your work, home, family, or school schedule of course but try to arrange something as close to this as possible.

If you schedule four to five hours or more in one day you are most likely defeating the purpose and wasting your time as your retention will start to decrease in hours three and beyond.

This is specially true if you have other commitments that require your time. Scheduling three or more hours of study time per day can actually add MORE stress to your life and reduce your sleeping time.

Either way this is exactly what you want to avoid at all costs! And I do mean ALL COSTS!

Scheduling time each day will keep you mentally fresh and absorbing good information PLUS it will give you the proper time for other commitments too! The outcome... reduce stressed.

Study With A Buddy

Whenever possible try to study with a buddy. Each person brings a different perspective to the learning process. This is a good way to retain new information because you are more focused on the task at hand when you are with someone else.

Plus, when you commit to study with a buddy the chances are you will actually follow through with your scheduled study time. No one likes to break a promise or commitment.

Commitment

Committing to study with a buddy is kind of like working out. It is hard to get motivated and push yourself to workout daily by yourself. That is just a fact. Only the most disciplined people can do this on their own and even some times they find it a challenge.

When you commit to meet a friend to workout it is much easier to keep your routine and commitment. Even though you may not want to workout that day, you recall the commitment you made to your friend and off you go to follow up on your commitment.

That commitment actually carries a lot of psychological weight with it. That is why people follow through with commitments made to others or in public and why it is important for you to commit to study with a buddy.

Plus the company never hurts either. Chances are you will both motivate each other to do more than you would have done alone.

The more you feel that you are not "in this alone" the more relaxed and confident you will be and the more you will get done.

Note: IMPORTANT**** *Study with a positive minded person. Don't get stuck listening to negative people and their excuses why they can't do this or that. These people are always looking to drag other people "down to their level" and are always reluctant to change to better themselves.*

If you arrange to study with a buddy and the person starts making negative comments... get out now! Don't waist your time trying to bring them up or convert them to your way of thinking.... it won't work! Stay positive and spend your time studying... not counseling. Leave that to the professionals.

Develop Your Concentration

Concentration is described as "intense mental application; complete attention".

It is your minds ability to focus on the task at hand and block out all other influences and distractions. To concentrate on one thing and one thing exclusively... the exam.

Information Retention

Your ability to concentrate is vital to your exam success. The more you concentrate on the subject materials the better you will retain and recall the information when the time comes to perform.

When you concentrate solely on the material it allows you less time to worry about other "stressors" or to give time for negative thoughts to enter in. And negative thoughts will try to work their way in. Self doubt is something that can be destructive so don't give your mind an opportunity to entertain negative thoughts.

For you to perform your best, all attention must be on the study material and the exam. This deep level of concentration will help you maximize your study time. In most cases, the better you can concentrate during your study time the less study time you will actually have to schedule. The saying "quality over quantity" applies to exam preparation too!

I mean... really, who wants to study for 5 hours at one sitting when you can study for 2 hours, with a high level of concentration and focus, and get the same results. No one. **Study Smarter, Not Longer!**

Benefits

Training your mind to concentrate on the task at hand will keep positive thoughts flowing and block out negative thoughts. Think of your mind as a bowl. You can only put so much in a bowl. So the more positive thoughts you put into the bowl the less room there is for negative ones.

Some of the benefits of increasing your level of concentration included:

• Peace of mind

• Self confidence

• Inner strength

• Ability to focus your mind

• Increased memory

• Ability to study and comprehend more quickly

• Less study time

Exercises

Here are some exercises to help you develop your concentration.

1) Select one thought and concentrate on it for ten minutes. This will be difficult at first but the more you do it the easier it will be to block out all other thoughts and concentrate on the one thought you have chosen.

2) Count the words in a paragraph. Count them again to ensure accuracy. Once you have completed this, count several paragraphs and then an entire page.

3) Take an object such as a spoon, fork, or anything out of a drawer. Try to concentrate on the object without mentally describing the object in words. Just focus on the object from all directions.

4) Draw a circle and color it in with any color. Now focus on the object and try not to think of any words, just focus on the object for several minutes.

5) Lie down and relax all your muscles. Once you are completely relaxed concentrated on your heartbeat and imagine your blood flowing throughout your body. After several minutes you should be able to feel the blood moving through your veins.

6) Watch the second hand on a clock. Focus just on the second hand and nothing else. Do this for two to three minutes and fight off the urge to let any other thoughts interfere with your concentration.

7) Close your eyes and visualize the number one. Say the number "one" in your head once you visualize it clearly. Now let it go and focus on the number two and repeat the process up to ten.

8) Take a coin out of your pocket. Relax every muscle in your body and concentrate on the coin and only the coin. View everything about it, its shape, color, material makeup nicks, words. Now close your eyes and visualize the coin in full detail. If you can not visualize the coin in full detail open your eyes and try again.

9) Sit in a chair and relax. Focus on a spot on the wall and release all other thoughts from your mind. Now while looking at the spot on the wall focus on your breathing. Breath in slowly and then exhale slowly. Do this for several minutes.

10) Read an article in the newspaper. Capture the essentials of the article. Now describe the article in as few words as possible to a friend or just aloud to yourself.

Learning to concentrate fully on the task at hand is difficult but the benefits are enormous. It is easy to let your mind wander off and loose your train of thought during an exam.

The better your concentration is during your exam preparation the better your exam scores will be. It is as simple as that.

Concentration is critical, specially towards the end of the exam when it is easy to get distracted and lose focus as you start to get tired.

This is when this training will pay off. You <u>will</u> remain focused and keep your concentration though the entire exam.

Note: IMPORTANT**** *These exercises are not for everyone, however, they are a valuable tool when learning to increase your concentration and mental focus.*

Try to do the exercises every other day. You will notice an increase in your information retention and recall. Plus this will help you study more efficiently and effectively!

Power of Positive Thinking

Positive thinking can reduce stress, improve your overall health, and make you much more interesting and fun to be around.

Although it is unclear exactly why positive thinkers experience health benefits, one of the theories is it helps them deal with stressful situations better. They are thinking of the best outcome, not the worst outcome, and this creates less stress and anxiety. This is better for the mind and the body.

I'll never forget an acquaintance of mine way back in the mid 80's who would shoot down new ideas like clay pigeons. Whenever a new idea would come up he would spend three times the intellectual effort to shoot it down than to consider if it would ever work. In his eyes "it would never work" no matter what it was.

Does that guy sound familiar to you? My guess is he probably does. You might have one or several people like this in your life right now. The best thing you can do is run... run... run.

I have nothing against shooting holes in a new idea to see if it stands the test of scrutiny, but just to dismiss a new idea because it represents change is unhealthy.

Negative people will try with all their might to bring you down. To make you surrender your positive "can do" attitude and keep them company in their pool of negativity. Don't let them!

Glass Half Full or Empty

Are you a "glass half full" or "glass half empty" type of person? Answering this question is a good way to find out if you are an optimist or a pessimist.

If you always see the good side of things (glass half full) then you are an optimist. If not, then you are a pessimist.

Optimists (or positive people) always consider the "what if it could work" side of things. They are happy and easy with a smile. They give as much positive energy as they get from others and are usually interesting and fun to be around.

An optimist is more likely to be successful too. They "will their self to victory". They tell THEMSELVES they can do something and this starts the ball of positivity and success rolling. Just as a snowball rolling down a mountain starts small, once it gains momentum there is little way to stop it.

Self Talk

Why is self talk important? Well, the mind is always thinking and creating "self-talk". Self-talk is the endless stream of thoughts that run through your head.

Self-talk is based on information, reason, logic, and prior experience. Self-talk also comes from misconceptions created because of misinformation or lack of information. This can be negative or positive, depending on your outlook.

For example, if someone asked you to jump over a hurdle and you've never jumped over a hurdle before, your mind would tell you either "you can do this" or "no way you can do this". This is commonly referred to as self-talk.

"PROGRAM THE VOICE INSIDE YOUR HEAD. IT WILL LISTEN, YOU OWN IT."

Programing your self talk will help you control the way you look at things and the attitude you have towards them. Self-talk is enormously powerful and you want to have it on your side.

A good example of the power of self-talk became apparent to me while working out several years ago and its power and control made a lasting impression on me.

In 1998 I started to lap swim at the local YMCA. I started to lap swim for several reasons. First, to lose weight that had accumulated over years of sitting behind a desk and remaining inactive. And second, to relieve some of the stress that comes with an upper level management job that I had been promoted to several years before.

The process of building up to a meaningful workout was slow at first, only a swimming a few laps per session. But over time I had built up to swimming 27 laps (which equalled 3/4 of a mile) per session.

I stayed at that level for many years, mainly because I could get my workout in over an hour long lunch break. But a funny thing happened several years ago when I finally went to work for myself. And it was all brought to light while talking to fellow lap swimmer at the local YMCA.

Through conversation she asked "how far do you swim each day". I said "3/4 of a mile". She asked, "why don't you just swim a mile"? "I don't know" I replied. "I have been doing this for years and never gave it much thought".

The next time in the pool I tried to swim a mile (36 laps) and around lap number twenty my mind began telling me I was tired and it was almost time to quit.

And sure enough, at lap twenty seven I was in no position to go any further. I was done. My mind had convinced my body that 3/4 of a mile was enough for today.

It was hard to believe that my body just started to feel exhausted around the 3/4 mile mark, knowing full well I could swim more laps. So the next day I decided to control my self-talk and tell myself "I am going to swim thirty six laps today" and "I could do anything I put my mind to". I was literally trying to trick myself into thinking I could swim a full mile.

Swimming a full mile was not a problem that day because my mind was reinforcing the belief that I could swim a mile. By controlling my self-talk and keeping the self-talk positive instead of negative I was able to control the outcome and achieve more than what my mind had previously programed me to accept as my unconscious limit.

I have also used this technique to swim two miles in one session and lose over 60 lbs. Controlling your self-talk is powerful, and it works.

Unconscious Limits

Your mind sets unconscious limits for everything that you do based on previous experience and other inputs of information such as things you read or discuss with others. Your mind processes all this information to set predetermined limits for you.

This was exceptionally powerful when world class runners were trying to break the four minute mile mark. It was generally thought that no one could ever run a mile under four minutes.

And for years no one could surpass that mark until May 6th, 1954. Sir Roger Bannister ran a mile in 3:59. Until that day no one had ever recorded running a mile under four minutes.

How strong was that unconscious limit? So strong that it only took **_46 days_** for the record to be broken. The unconscious limit had been stripped away, and in only 46 days another runner achieved what only one man had ever achieved before. The sub four minute mile.

The same applies to your exam preparation. Remove your unconscious limits and give your mind the freedom to perform the way it is capable of. Learning to channel self-talk in a positive direction can help you achieve more than you ever imagined.

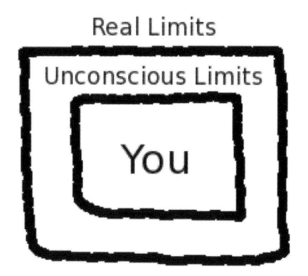

Train Your Mind

In the end, the mind will do what you <u>train</u> it to do. For example, do you ever catch yourself saying subconsciously that you *can't* do something? Of course you have. We all have. That is because we haven't trained our minds to accept the challenge of the task we want to perform.

It is our job to change the way we think. Think positive thoughts. "I CAN do this". "I am the best". "I <u>will</u> pass the exam". Train your mind to think positively and this will reduce your stress level and give you a confident feeling going into the exam.

Do not let others, or your surroundings, dictate your mental state of mind. <u>YOU</u> have the ultimate control and <u>YOU</u> control whether you think positive or negative thoughts.

This takes time and it is something that should be practiced daily. Do not think you can think positive once and everything will occur as you would like it. It just doesn't work that way. Even when you fail, resist the urge to be negative. Everything worthwhile takes some effort. But over time this will work in your favor.

You have to remember you are potentially trying to undo years of "I CAN"T" programming. Years of people telling you "YOU CAN'T" and "NO" and "IT WILL NEVER WORK".

Those are powerful messages built in to your mind. We have all heard them for many years and now is the time to turn it around.

The first "YES I CAN", and "I CAN DO WHATEVER I PUT MY MIND TO" will begin the change. It will start the little snowball rolling down the mountain... and with a little momentum comes massive change!

Self Confidence

Confidence shows in everything you do. From how you look at life to how you treat others. Confident people are people who take action. Confident people are the "doers" in the world. The people who look for ways for things to work rather than look for ways for things to fail.

Confidence is not arrogance. Confidence comes from taking decisive action and not from the outcome of that action. Confident people do not shy away from taking action because they are afraid of a failed outcome. They take action and are undaunted by the prospect of failure.

Arrogance, however, is exactly the opposite. Arrogance does not come from taking action, it comes from the result of the action. Arrogance highlights achievements and hides failures never learning anything from either.

An arrogant person is defined, in their own mind, by both their accomplishments and failures and will shy away from taking action because of the prospect of failure.

Developing Confidence

Confidence is developed through a series of "wins" or "achievements". It is developed through facing your fears and overcoming them. This gives you strength and confidence in your ability to overcome. The more you overcome, the more confident you become.

So how do you build confidence in your ability to pass an exam? Simple.... preparation! Face your fears head on and take action. Prepare every day until you know you are going to pass... there is not doubt!

Review the study material over and over again and build your level of confidence. There is no substitute for hard work and hard work builds confidence.

Have you ever seen a person walk into a room and everyone pays attention? They have a certain confidence about them that radiates form within.

They are not the wealthiest in the room. Nor the most attractive person. But this inner confidence puts them at ease when everyone else may be timid or afraid to step out of their comfort zone.

Confidence and the Exam

Your confidence will have a direct effect on your exam results. If you are confident in your ability to pass the exam it lowers your stress level and opens your mind for clearer thinking. When you project confidence your body reacts differently to circumstances. It gives you the calmness to perform at a high level.

Confidence only comes through preparation. The more you prepare, the more confident you will be in your ability to ace your exam.
This is the type of confidence you must have when you walk into the exam. An undeniable belief that you will pass the exam because of your preparation, determination, and hard work.

Nothing will stand in your way from achieving your goal!

"YOU GAIN STRENGTH, COURAGE AND CONFIDENCE BY EVERY EXPERIENCE IN WHICH YOU STOP TO LOOK FEAR IN THE FACE. YOU ARE ABLE TO SAY TO YOURSELF, 'I HAVE LIVED THROUGH THIS HORROR. I CAN TAKE THE NEXT THING THAT COMES ALONG.' YOU MUST DO THE THING YOU THINK YOU CANNOT DO."

ELEANOR ROOSEVELT

Sleep and Nutrition

The final piece of the puzzle to reducing stress is proper sleep and nutrition. Your body and mind can only function at its highest level if you give it proper rest and proper nutrition (fuel).

Your body and mind needs time to rest and good food to perform. This is easy to overlook and many times it is the first thing you sacrifice when you are preparing for an exam.

You can do everything else right to reduce stress and prepare for an exam but failing to get proper rest and nutrition could cause it all to go to waste.

Once you think about it you can see why these are essential ingredients (no pun intended) to successful exam preparation.

Sleep

Why is sleep so important? Because it is the only time your body has a chance to recharge.

A good sleep regiment should consist of at least six hours of sleep each night so your body and mind are fresh and ready to go the next morning. Anything less an you will not be fully rested and your performance will suffer because of it.

Stress can also impact sleep patterns to a point that is unhealthy. Stress related sleep disorders are fairly common and can have a major impact on your exam performance.

How many times have you tried to solve work or family related problems well into the night. Sometimes it just cannot be avoided but trying to leave work at work and going to bed with a clear mind will leave you refreshed and ready to tackle the problems of the day when the next day arrives.

To get a better nights sleep try these simple tips to reduce stress and rest up.

1) List problems bothering you with possible solutions before bed.

2) Put work into perspective. When work is over, leave it. Turn it off.

3) Designate cell free time. Even if it is only a half hour or during dinner.

4) Never check work email before bed.

5) Try to simplify one thing each day.

6) Grab a nap if you can. Sleep reduces stress hormones.

7) Laugh! Laughter reduces stress and raises <u>anti-stress</u> hormones making it easier to fall asleep.

8) Owning a pets can significantly lower your heart rate and blood pressure letting you rest longer.

9) Hug a family member. Affection reduces stress and makes it easier to sleep.

10) Take a fifteen minute walk. Exercise is the <u>BEST</u> stress reliever and you will be ready to sleep when the time comes!

These tips can make it easier to get a good nights rest and ready to go in the morning.

Nutrition

Proper nutrition to reduce stress you say? Yes, it's true! Proper nutrition plays a key role in our body's performance and ability to rest.

There is plenty of information about the ties between nutrition and sleep. One of my favorite articles is called "Sleep Deeper with Better Nutrition". It covers a mound of information about protein "super foods" and herbs that will help you get a better nights rest naturally.

Some of the "super foods" are items such as green tea, buffalo, walnuts, sardines, artichokes, kiwis, dark chocolate, cherries, and many others. These foods supply the body with super fuel and burn very efficiently so you don't feel full or tired after eating them.

I prefer making adjustments to diet over prescription drugs or other methods because it is natural and enhances the body's ability to rest.

Food or drink that contain sugar or caffeine can give you a temporary boost but the crash won't help you towards the end of the exam when you typically need it the most so try to avoid these.

What If I Fail?

The most successful people fail all the time! It is a result of taking action. There is no shame in failure, only shame in not getting back up, learning from your mistakes, and trying again.

Golf legend Jack Nicklaus used to welcome a bad golf hole or two each round because the sooner he got them out of the way the sooner he could move on and make the round a great one. He embraced temporary failure as part of being successful.

Truthfully, the more you fail the closer you are to succeeding as long as you learn from your mistakes. Few people succeed without failing many times first. It's a learning process and failure is one of the steps. You can say failure is the downpayment on success and it really is. Chances are good you will fail before you succeed but don't let it define you or hold you back. Expect it and learn from it. If you don't fail it shows you haven't taken action and just sat on the sidelines and that is the worst fate of all.

Overcome your fear of failure and success will be yours. Nothing will stand in your way. Preparation is the key. If you have prepared properly you will not fail. But if you should, embrace it, be accountable for it, and start again with more resolve than ever.

The highway is littered with people who have failed. Everyone fails. The people who win get right back on the horse and start riding again.

"I HAVE NOT FAILED. I'VE JUST FOUND 10,000 WAYS THAT WON'T WORK."

THOMAS EDISON

Getting Help

Is there a certain section of material that is just not making sense or sinking in? GET HELP! Don't wait or, worse yet, be too shy to ask for help. Search out help as fast as you can. Now is not the time to be shy or hesitate to ask for assistance.

Many teachers and instructors are more than willing to give you a helping hand. That is their profession and most of them generally love to help people. Take advantage of their help if you need it.

REMEMBER, YOU ARE NOT IN THIS ALONE!

Reaching out for help and getting it will give you a feeling of accomplishment and confidence. That confidence will be your friend and something you want to continually build upon as you ready yourself for your exam.

"ONE IMPORTANT KEY TO SUCCESS IS SELF-CONFIDENCE. AN IMPORTANT KEY TO SELF- CONFIDENCE IS PREPARATION."

ARTHUR ASHE

Common Anatomical Terminology

Anatomy terminology can seem complex and overwhelming when just starting out. Once you familiarize yourself with some of the more common terms it will make your preparation much easier. Just like anything else, it will take practice. Learn and few terms each day and before you know it you will have established a good base to work from.

Take time to familiarize yourself with these terms to make you a better medical coder.

Anatomy Terminology - Number	
Term	**Meaning**
mono-, uni-	one
bi	two
tri	three

Anatomy Terminology - Direction and Position	
Term	**Meaning**
ab-	away from
ad-	toward
ecto-, exo-	outside
endo-	inside
epi-	upon
anterior or ventral	at or near the front surface of the body
posterior or dorsal	at or near the real surface of the body
superior	above
inferior	below
lateral	side
distal	farthest from center
proximal	nearest to center

Anatomy Terminology - Basic Terms	
Term	**Meaning**
abdominal	abdomen
buccal	cheek
cranial	skull
digital	fingers and toes
femoral	thigh
gluteal	buttocks
hallux	great toe
inguinal	groin
lumbar	lowest part of spine
mammary	breast
nasal	nose
occipital	back of head
pectoral	breastbone
thoracic	chest
umbilical	navel
ventral	belly

Anatomy Terminology - Conditions - Prefixes	
Term	**Meaning**
ambi-	both
dys-	bad, painful, difficult
eu-	good, normal
homo-	same
iso-	equal, same
mal-	bad, poor

Anatomy Terminology - Conditions - Suffixes	
Term	**Meaning**
-algia	pain
-emia	blood
-itis	inflammation
-lysis	destruction, breakdown
-oid	like
-opathy	disease of
-pnea	breathing

Anatomy Terminology - Surgical Procedures	
Term	**Meaning**
-centesis	puncture a cavity to remove fluid
-ectomy	surgical removal or excision
-ostomy	a new permanent opening
-otomy	cutting into, incision
-opexy	surgical fixation
-oplasty	surgical repair
-otripsy	crushing or destroying

Medical Terminology Prefix, Root, and Suffixes

Being familiar with Medical Terminology prefixes, roots and suffixes are essential for a medical coder. This illustrates how roots, prefixes, and suffixes are used to denote number or size, direction, color, anatomical locations, as well as other meanings.

Medical Terminology - Prefixes and Roots Denoting Number or Size	
Term	**Meaning**
bi-	two
dipl/o	two, double
hemi-	half
hyper-	over or more than usual
hypo-	under or less than usual
iso-	equal, same
macro-	large
megal/o-	enlargement
micro-	small
mono-	one
multi-	many
nulli-	none
poly-	many
semi-	half, partial
tri-	three
uni-	one

| Medical Terminology - Roots Denoting Color ||
Term	Meaning
chlor/o	green
cyan/o	blue
erythr/o	red
leuk/o	white
melan/o	black
xanth/o	yellow

Medical Terminology - Prefixes and Roots Denoting Relative Direction	
Term	**Meaning**
per-	through
peri-	around
post-	behind, after
poster/o	behind
pre-	before, in front of
pro-	before
retr/o	behind, in back of
sub-	under
super-	beyond
supra-	above
syn-	together
trans-	across
ventr/o	belly

Medical Terminology - Roots Denoting Anatomical Location	
Term	**Meaning**
abdomin/o	abdomen
acr/o	extremity
aden/o	gland
angi/o	vessel
arter/i/o	artery
arthr/o	joint
blast/o	embryo
blephar/o	eyelid
bronch/i/o	bronchus
calcane/o	calaneous
cardi/o	heart
carp/o	carpal, wrist
cephal/o	head
cerebr/o	cerebrum
cheil/o	lip
chol/e	bile, gall
chondr/o	cartilage
cocc/i	coccus
col/o	colon
colp/o	vagina

Medical Terminology - Roots Denoting Anatomical Location

Term	Meaning
condyl/o	condyle
core/o, cor/o	pupil
corne/o	cornea
cost/o	ribs
crani/o	cranium
cycl/o	ciliary body
cyst/o	bladder, sac
cyt/o	cell
dactyl/o	fingers or toes
dent/o	tooth
derm/o	skin
dermat/o	skin
duoden/o	duodenum
enter/o	intestine
esophag/o	esophagus
fibr/o	fiber
gangli/o	ganglion
gastr/o	stomach
gingiv/o	gums
gloss/o	tongue

Medical Terminology - Roots Denoting Anatomical Location	
Term	**Meaning**
gynec/o	women
hem/o, hemat/o	blood
hepat/o	liver
hidr/o	sweat
humer/o	humerus
hydr/o	water
hyster/o	uterus
ile/o	ileum
irid/o, ir/o	iris
ischi/o	ischium
jejun/o	jejunum
kerat/o	cornea
lacrim/o	tear
laryng/o	larynx
lip/o	fat
lith/o	stone, calculus
lumb/o	loin, lumbar area
ment/o	chin
my/o	muscle
myel/o	spinal cord, bone marrow

| Medical Terminology - Roots Denoting Anatomical Location ||
Term	Meaning
nas/o	nose
nephr/o	kidney
neur/o	nerve
omphal/o	umbilicus, navel
onych/o	nail
oophor/o	ovary
opthalm/o	eye
orchid/o	testicles
oste/o	bone
ot/o	ear
pancreat/o	pancreas
pely/i	pelvis
peps/o/ia	digestion
phalang/o	phalange
pharyng/o	pharynx
phas/o	speech
phleb/o	veins
pleur/o	pleura
pne/o	air, breathing
pneum/o, pneumono	lung

Medical Terminology - Roots Denoting Anatomical Location

Term	Meaning
pod/o	foot
proct/o	rectum, anus
psych/o	mind
pub/o	pubis
py/o	pus
pyel/o	kidney
rect/o	rectum
ren/o	kidney
retin/o	retina
rhin/o	nose
salping/o	fallopian tube
scler/o	sclera
spermat/o	sperm
splen/o	spleen
stern/o	sternum, breastbone
stomat/o	mouth
thorac/o	thorax, chest
trache/o	trachea
traumat/o	tramua
tympan/o	eardrum

Medical Terminology - Roots Denoting Anatomical Location	
Term	**Meaning**
ur/o	urine
ureter/o	ureter
urethr/o	urethra
vas/o	vessel
viscer/o	gut, contents of the abdomen

Medical Terminology - Other Prefixes	
Term	**Meaning**
a-, an-	without
anti-	against
auto-	self
brady-	slow
con-	with
contra-	against
dis-	free of
dys-	difficult or without pain
mal-	bad, poor
neo-	new
syn-	together
tachy-	fast

Medical Terminology - Other Roots	
Term	**Meaning**
necr/o	dead
noct/i	night
par/o	bear
phag/o	eat
phil/o	attraction
plast/o	repair, formation
pyr/o	fire, fever
scler/o	tough, hard
sinistr/o	left
syphil/o	syphilis
therap/o	treatment
therm/o	heat
thromb/o	thrombosis
troph/o	development

Medical Terminology - Other Suffixes

Term	Meaning
algia	pain
ar	pertaining to
centesis	puncture
clysis	irrigation
ectasia	dilatation, dilation
ectomy	excision
emes/is	vomiting
emia	blood
esthesia	feelings
genesis, gen/o	development, formation, beginning
gnosis	know
ia	noun ending
ia, ic	pertaining to
it is	inflammation
manual	hand
meter	measuring instrument
oid	resembling
ologist	one who studies
ology	study of
oma	tumor

Medical Terminology - Other Suffixes	
Term	**Meaning**
opia	vision
orrhagia	hemorrhage
orrhaphy	suture
orrhea	flow
orrhexis	rupture
osis	condition of
ostomy	new opening
otomy	incision
pedal	foot
pexy	fixing, fixation
phob/ia	fear
plasm	growth
plegia, plegic	paralysis
ptosis	drooping
scope, scopy	examining, looking at
spasm	twitching
sperm	sperm
stasis	slow, stop
tome	instrument
tripsy	crushing

Notes

Resources

Exam Preparation Products We Recommend

Medical Coding Exam Prep Course
http://medicalcodingpro.com/medical-coding-certification-prep-course/

Medical Coding Exam System
http://medicalcodingexamsystem.com

Faster Coder - Code Faster - Code Better
http://fastercoder.com

Other Resources

Elite Members Area – 7 day FREE trial!
http://medicalcodingpromembers.com

Medical Coding Pro – main website
http://medicalcodingpro.com

MEDICAL CODING PRO

Medical Coding Pro provides information about medical coding. We also help people in the medical coding community prepare for the medical coding certification exam.

Our mission is to help everyone we can pass the exam and gain their certification as quickly as possible.To do this we offer quality exam preparation tools such as Medical Coding Practice Exams, the Medical Coding Exam System, the Medical Coding Exam Strategy and the Medical Coding Pro Elite Members Area.

Visit us on the web at:

www.MedicalCodingPro.com

www.MedicalCodingProMembers.com

www.MedicalCodingExamSystem.com

www.MedicalCodingNews.org

Made in the USA
San Bernardino, CA
27 April 2019